Official Journal of the Internatior
Blood Purification

Blood Purification

Founded 1983; edited by K. Schaefer (1983–1988)

KARGER

Printed in Switzerland
on acid-free paper by
Thür AG Offsetdruck, Pratteln

Appears bimonthly:
1 volume per year (6 issues)

Submission: Only original papers written in English are considered and should be sent to:

S. Karger AG
Editorial Dept. 'Blood Purification'
P.O. Box
CH-4009 Basel (Switzerland)

Manuscripts should be submitted in quadruplicate (with four sets of illustrations of which one is an original), typewritten double-spaced on one side of the paper, with a wide margin.

Conditions: All manuscripts are subject to editorial review. Manuscripts are received with the explicit understanding that they are not under simultaneous consideration by any other publication. Submission of an article for publication implies the transfer of the copyright from the author to the publisher upon acceptance. Accepted papers become the permanent property of 'Blood Purification' and may not be reproduced by any means, in whole or in part, without the written consent of the publisher. It is the author's responsibility to obtain permission to reproduce illustrations, tables, etc. from other publications.

Arrangement:
Title page: The first page of each paper should indicate the title (main title underlined), the authors' names, and the institute where the work was conducted. A short title for use as running head as well as the full address of the author to whom correspondence should be sent are also required.
Full address: The exact postal address complete with postal code must be given at the bottom of the title page. Please also supply Phone, Fax, and E-mail numbers.
Key words: For indexing purposes, a list of 3–10 key words in English is essential.
Abstract: Each paper needs an abstract of up to 10 lines.
Small type: Paragraphs which can or must be set in smaller type (case histories, test methods, etc.) should be indicated with a 'p' (petit) in the margin on the left-hand side.
Footnotes: Avoid footnotes. When essential, they are numbered consecutively and typed at the foot of the appropriate page.
Tables and illustrations: Tables and illustrations (both numbered in Arabic numerals) should be prepared on separate sheets. Tables require a heading and figures a legend, also prepared on a separate sheet. For the reproduction of illustrations, only good drawings and original photographs can be accepted; negatives or photocopies cannot be used. When possible, group several illustrations on one block for reproduction (max. size 140 × 188 mm) or provide crop marks. On the back of each illustration, indicate its number, the author's name, and 'top'.

Color illustrations: Up to 6 color illustrations per page can now be integrated with the text at the reduced price of SFr. 600.–/US$ 545.00 per page. Color illustrations are reproduced at the author's expense.

References: In the text identify references by Arabic numerals [in square brackets]. Material submitted for publication but not yet accepted should be noted as 'unpublished data' and not be included in the reference list. The list of references should include only those publications which are cited in the text. Do not alphabetize; number references in the order in which they are first mentioned in the text. The surnames of the authors followed by initials should be given. There should be no punctuation other than a comma to separate the authors. Cite all authors, 'et al' is not sufficient. Abbreviate journal names according to the Index Medicus system. (Also see International Committee of Medical Journal Editors: Uniform requirements for manuscripts submitted to biomedical journals. Br Med J 1988;296: 401–405.)
Examples
(a) Papers published in periodicals: Kauffman HF, van der Heide S, Beaumont F, Blok H, de Vries K: Class-specific antibody determination against *Aspergillus fumigatus* by means of the enzyme-linked immunosorbent assay. III. Comparative study: IgG, IgA, IgM ELISA titers, precipitating antibodies and IgE binding after fractionation of the antigen. Int Arch Allergy Appl Immunol 1986;80:300–306.
(b) Monographs: Matthews DE, Farewell VT: Using and Understanding Medical Statistics. Basel, Karger, 1985.
(c) Edited books: Hardy WD Jr, Essex M: FeLV-induced feline acquired immune deficiency syndrome: A model for human AIDS; in Klein E (ed): Acquired Immunodeficiency Syndrome. Prog Allergy. Basel, Karger, 1986, vol 37, pp 353–376.
Further details: Authors may consult our leaflet 'Rules for the Preparation of Manuscripts', available on request from the Publisher, S. Karger AG, P.O. Box, CH-4009 Basel (Switzerland).

Rapid communication: Manuscripts intended for rapid communication must present new findings of sufficient importance to justify their accelerated acceptance. They should follow the general arrangement of research papers except that the separate sections should not be formally titled. They should not be more than three pages in length (including figures, tables and references). Proofs are checked by the Managing Editor and not sent to the authors. Review will be rapid, and once accepted, the paper will be included in the next planned issue.

Page charges: There is no page charge for papers of 4 or fewer printed pages (including tables, illustrations and references). Each additional complete or partial page is charged to the author at SFr. 245.– / US $ 196.00. The allotted size of a paper is equal to approx. 7 manuscript pages (including tables, illustrations and references).

Galley proofs: Unless indicated otherwise, galley proofs are sent to the first-named author and should be returned with the least possible delay. Alterations made in galley proofs, other than the correction of printer's errors, are charged to the author. No page proofs are supplied.

Reprints: Order forms and a price list are sent with the galley proofs. Orders submitted after the issue is printed are subject to considerably higher prices. Allow five weeks from date of publication for delivery of reprints.

KARGER

13th Annual Meeting of the International Society of Blood Purification

Abstracts

September 27–29, 1995
Kyongju, Korea

Guest Editors
Hi Bahl Lee, Seoul
Han Chul Park, Seoul

KARGER

Blood Purification

Vol. 13, Supplement 1, 1995

Sponsors of the XIIIth Annual Meeting of The International Society of Blood Purification

The Korean Society of Nephrology
The Korean Medical Association
Ministry of Health and Welfare
Korea Science and Engineering Foundation
Korea Research Foundation
Korea Tourism National Corporation
Honorable Mr. Hwang Yoon Ki, Member of the National Assembly
City of Kyongju
Kolon Industries, Inc.
Boryung Pharmaceutical Co., Ltd.
Gambro Group
Baxter Healthcare Corporation
Korea Green Cross Medical Corp.
Choongwae Pharmaceutical Co., Ltd.
Saejin Medicare Corp. / COBE
Myongmoon Pharmaceutical Co., Ltd.
Baxter Korea Incorporated
Fresenius AG
Gambro Asia
Gambro Korea
Akzo Nobel
Boehringer Mannheim
Nishho Companies
Hanmi Pharmaceutical Co., Ltd.
Sandoz Pharma Ltd.

S. Karger
Medical and Scientific Publishers
Basel · Freiburg · Paris · London
New York · New Delhi · Bangkok
Singapore · Tokyo · Sydney

Drug Dosage
The authors and the publisher have exerted every effort to ensure that drug selection and dosage set forth in this text are in accord with current recommendations and practice at the time of publication. However, in view of ongoing research, changes in government regulations, and the constant flow of information relating to drug therapy and drug reactions, the reader is urged to check the package insert for each drug for any change in indications and dosage and for added warnings and precautions. This is particularly important when the recommended agent is a new and/or infrequently employed drug.

Printed in Korea by Medical Publishing Co.
ISBN 3-8055-6239-X

Foreword

Contained in this Supplement issue are 104 abstracts to be presented by scientists from 18 countries at the XIIIth Annual Meeting of the International Society of Blood Purification (ISBP), Kyongju, Korea, September 27-29, 1995.

Eleven abstracts will be presented at 3 Symposia : 1) Viral hepatitis in dialysis patients, 2) Medical applications of polymer materials, 3) Nutrition in dialysis patients.

The ISBP Annual Award Lecture is delivered by Professor Sung Wan Kim of University of Utah, Salt Lake City, USA and the title is Design of nonthrombogenic polymer surfaces for blood contacting medical devices.

The remaining abstracts are presented at free communication sessions, 3 oral and 5 simultaneous poster presentation session which cover a diverse areas of interests : 1) Techniques and results of removal of endogenous metabolites and exogenous toxic substances, 2) Biocompatibility of membranes, catheters, and dialysates, 3) Peritoneal and vascular access, 4) Nutrition and membrane transport physiology and pathology, 5) Immunomodulation, 6) Vascular reactivity and other clinical topics.

The discussions and exchange of informations that will follow the scientific presentations will undoubtedly stimulate the research in the field of blood purification by scientists from around the world. We hope, in the end, that all participants will have gained from the meeting, scientifically and socially.

Hi Bahl Lee, M.D.
Han Chul Park, M.D.
Guest Editors

Contents

General Information

Blood Purification

Publication data: 'Blood Purification' is published 6 times annually. Volume 13 with 6 issues appears in 1995.

Subscription rates: Subscriptions run for a full calendar year. Prices are given per volume.

Personal subscription:

Subscription	*+ postage and handling*
SFr. 300.30	+ SFr. 17.90 Europe
SFr. 300.30	+ SFr. 27.30 Overseas
US$ 231.00	+ US$ 17.90

(Must be in the name of, billed to, and paid by an individual. Order must be marked 'personal subscription'.)

Institutional subscription:

Subscription	*+ postage and handling*
SFr. 429.–	+ SFr. 25.50 Europe
SFr. 429.–	+ SFr. 39.– Overseas
US$ 330.00	+ US$ 25.50

Airmail postage: SFr. 36.–, US$ 30.00. (Extra per volume.)

Discount subscription prices:
International Society of Blood Purification

Microforms: Please direct all enquiries and orders to:
University Microfilms Inc.
300 North Zeeb Road, P.O. Box 1346
Ann Arbor, MI 48106-1346 (USA)

Subscription orders: Orders can be placed at agencies, bookstores, directly with the Publisher S. Karger AG, P.O. Box, CH – 4009 Basel (Switzerland) or with any of the following distributors:

Deutschland: S. Karger GmbH, Postfach
D – 79095 Freiburg

France: Librairie Luginbühl
36, bd de Latour-Maubourg
F-75007 Paris

Great Britain, Ireland: S. Karger Publishers
11 Ravenscroft Road
Beckenham, Kent BR3 4TP

USA: S. Karger Publishers, Inc.
26 West Avon Road, P.O. Box 529
Farmington, CT 06085

India, Bangladesh, Sri Lanka:
S. Karger India Subscription Agency
B – 5/132 Safdarjung Enclave
New Delhi-110029

Japan: Katakura Libri, Inc.
36-9 Hongo 3-chome, Bunkyo-ku
Tokyo 113

Change of address: Both old and new address should be sent to the subscription source.

Single issues and back volumes: Information can be obtained through the Publisher.

Advertising: Correspondence and rate requests should be addressed to the Publisher.

Bibliographic indices: This journal is regularly listed in bibliographic services, including *Current Contents®*.

Book Reviews: Books are accepted for review by special agreement.

Guidelines for Disk Submission

Karger Publishers welcomes the submission of manuscripts on disk.
Please observe the 'Instructions to Authors' as well as the following guidelines:

Technical Data

Storage medium is a 3.5- or 5.25-inch disk.
The preferred word processing package is Word for Windows®. Other commonly used PC text programs are also accepted, as well as ASCII formats.
MacIntosh® is also acceptable. However **1,44 Byte HD** in ASCII is preferred.

Handling

All manuscripts accepted for Karger publications are subject to copy-editing. It is therefore essential that you send us a **double-spaced printout** of your manuscript which exactly matches the disk.

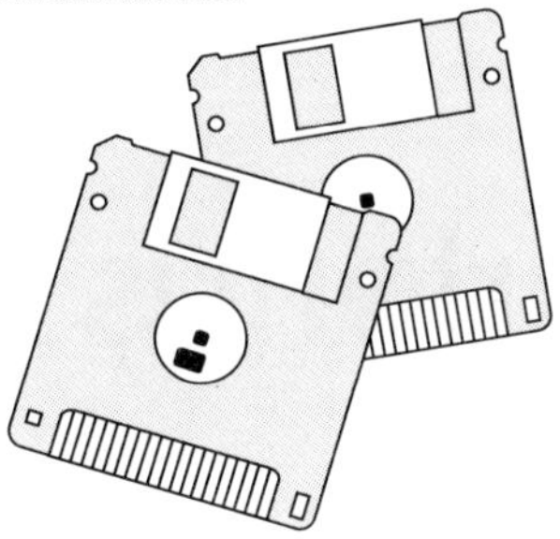

Any subsequent revised versions should be clearly marked as such, both on the disk and on the manuscript.
The copy-edited manuscript and the disk will be returned to you along with the galley proofs. Please be sure to **check the galleys against the manuscript** in which changes introduced by the copy-editor and/or questions will be marked.
Please **label** your disk with (a) the title of the journal or book for which it is submitted, (b) a short version of the paper title, (c) your name, (d) the software and hardware used and (e) the file names contained.
Do not place more than one article in a file.

Text Arrangement

Please follow the general rules about style given in the 'Instructions to Authors' or 'Rules for the Preparation of Manuscripts'.
Be sure to use the same type style for headings of the same ranking throughout the text. Be consistent and stick to the same work pattern throughout the manuscript.
Do not use automatic page numbering. Number the pages by hand.
Text and headings should be ranged left throughout, without word breaks. **Do not center, space, or use block letters** for text and headings (except for abbreviations). Do not split words (neither by hand nor automatically).
Do not use indentations anywhere in the manuscript, including the references. To mark the beginning of a paragraph, leave one blank line between paragraphs. Do not use a hyphenating program. Use the possibilities of your text program to emphasize text parts, e.g. **Bold,** *Italic,* $_{\text{Sub-}}$ and ^{Superscript}.
Insert one (and only one) space after each interpunctuation mark – e.g. at the end of sentences and with reference numbers, i.e. [22, 27, 35].
When using **special characters** not available on a standard keyboard (including Greek characters) please do so by a readily identifiable code, and use the same code throughout the manuscript. Supply a **complete list of the codes used** at the beginning of the text or include a 'Read-me-file'.
Do not use spaces in tables; use the tabulator. Operation data within tables (e.g. 15.1 ± 7.23) should be formatted in one column, not split into two.
Illustrations and mathematical formulae will be handled conventionally.

KARGER

Over 10,000 filtration systems installed worldwide – profit from Sartorius' extensive know-how

Working together with you, we design customized separation systems for the following application areas:
- Sterile filtration
- Clarification
- Filtration of air and other gases
- Crossflow filtration

The large number of filtration systems currently in operation throughout the world is proof of Sartorius' worldwide reputation for customer satisfaction and long years of engineering experience in filtration.

Implementation

Implementation means more than just supplying you with a product. At Sartorius, we offer a complete performance package that includes the following services:
- Commissioning
- Validation support
- Instruction and training of your staff
- Maintenance service

The system you purchase from Sartorius can be easily integrated into your process and quickly adapted to meet new operating conditions. Just ask us – we'll be glad to help you.

The right filtration process for your application

Sartorius systems are custom-engineered to optimally meet your individual needs. Each system features a modular design that uses only the most reliable of field-proven components. Based on your specifications, we scale and design your system by incorporating the components and interfaces that currently exist at your facilities.

Sartorius filtration systems feature on-screen monitoring of your entire process. This makes it easy to integrate them into new or existing processes and into process control systems. As a result, you avoid problems with interfacing. By working in close cooperation with you, we design filtration systems that have the utmost degree of cost-efficiency and process security.

Maximum profitability for complex filtration applications

The decisive criteria for profitability are:
- High yield
- Operating costs
- Return on investment (ROI)

To best meet these criteria, we conduct extensive testing on-site using pilot systems.

Sartorius' Delivery Service and Logistics Center assure smooth-running and profitable operations as well as low inventory costs.

List of References and Applications

Formulated Solutions	Bristol Myers Squibb, Italy	Pfizer, France	Glaxo, U.K.
Vaccines	Commonwealth Serum Laboratory (CSL), Australia	Pasteur Mérieux Sérums et Vaccins (PMSV), France	Evans Medical, U.K.
Blood Products	Pharmacia AB, Sweden	Miles/Bayer, USA	Speywood Biopharm, U.K.
Fermentation	Monico Jacopo, Italy	Smith Kline Beecham, USA	Boehringer Mannheim GmbH, Germany
Cell Cultures	Sanofi, France	Wellcome Beckenham, U.K.	Dr. Karl Thomae GmbH, Germany
Diagnostics	Kodak Diagnostics, U.K.	Cortecs Diagnostics, U.K.	

		Abstracts No.
Koda Y, Miyazaki S, Yuasa Y, Suzuki M, Hirasawa Y, Morita T, Kamura T Japan	Iliopsoas Bursitis is a Rare Complication Associated with BETA-2 Microglobulin (B2M) Amyloid in Long-term Hemodialysis Patients	**52**
Jo SK, Kwon YJ, Kim NH, Chang MK, Wee KS, Koo JR, Cha DR, Cho WY, Pyo HJ, Kim HK Korea	Pseudomonas Peritonotis in Patients on CAPD	**53**
Liou SY, Lin MP, Chang CL, Chen TJ Taiwan	Endotoxin Contamination in Reverse Osmosis -treated Water and Dialysate - A Multi Center Study	**54**
Chen XM, Liao HJ China	Effect of Epimedium Sagittatum on Quality of Life and Cellular Immunity in Patients on Maintained Hemodialysis	**55**
Chen XM, Zhu N China	Evaluation of the Dialytic Efficiency by KT/V Urea Modelling in High-Flux Hemodialysis (HFD)	**56**
Zhou MH, Chen XM China	A Survey of the Nutritional Status of Patients Undergoing Chronic Hemodialysis	**57**
Liao HJ, Chen XM, Liu SW China	Expression of Interleukin 8 (IL-8), IL-l beta and IL-6 mRNA in Hemodialysis (HD) Patients	**58**
Chen XM, Zhu N China	Biocompatibility of Dialyser Membranes: Comparision of Four Kinds of Hemodialysis Membranes	**59**
Marangoni R, Savino R, Masi F, Manfredi A, Cimino R, Colombo R, Maltagliati L, Longhena GR Italia	B2 Microglobulin (B2-M) Removal with Different Blood Purification Extracorporeal Methods	**60**
Benedik M, Ponikvar R, Guček A, Varl J, Buturović-Ponikvar J, Kveder R, Merc J Slovenia	The Elimination of Vitamin D with CAPD Fluid is Important in CAPD Patients	**61**
Kim H, Kim KT, Chon YC, Lee SJ, Lee EJ, Park SE, Suh SY, Kim SS, Cha DR, Koo JR, Kwon YJ, Cho WY, Kim HK Korea	Prevalence of Anti-HCV Antibody in Chronic Hemodialysis Patients (multi-center study)	**62**
Kang SK, Lee KS, Kim JH, Koh JK, Park SK Korea	Endotoxin Level in Dialysis Systems	**63**
Hillion D, Haas T, Savoiu C, Elbouatmani A, Uzan M, Pertuiset N France	Which Membrane for Predilution HF?	**64**
Haas T, Hillion D, Guerrito MJ, Robine M, Uzan M, Pertuiset N France	No Relationship Between Increase in Extracoporeal Clearances and Small Molecules Mass Removal	**65**

1

Renal Replacement Therapy in The Critically Ill

CD Scheinkestel, P.S. Myles, D.V. Tuxen, D.J. Cooper

Alfred Hospital, Melbourne, Australia

Renal failure occurred in 10.1% of 4140 patients in a tertiary referral ICU over 8 years. 140 patients (3.4%) received renal replacement therapies. 94% of these had 3 organ system failures.

Results. (1) Increased ICU stay (and cost) in dialysed vs non-dialysed patients. (18 vs 5.7 days: $p = 0.00001$; US $10,170). (2) Overall survival rate of 41%, 34% for $\geq$ 3 OSFs and 18% for 7 OSFs are better than previously reported by Knaus (34% vs 20%, $p = 0.01$). (3) Apache 2 predicted risk of death matched actual mortality (55% vs 59%; NS), but was a poor predictor of outcome in individuals (p = NS). (4) Best predictors of outcome were the number of OSF (odds ratio 2.34, $p = 0.00005$) and age > 65 (odds ratio: 2.5, $p = 0.044$) but neither were predictive in the individual. (5) Survivors had significantly lower OSFs (5 ± 2 vs 6 ± 1: $p = 0.0005$) and Apache 2 scores (26 vs 28 $p = 0.04$). There was no difference in sex, age or diagnostic category. ICU length of stay was longer for survivors compared to non-survivors. (21 ± 22 vs 16 ± 13: $p = 0.001$). (6) At hospital discharge, 51% of survivors recovered baseline renal function, 33% had significant deterioration and 16% deterioration to endstage disease or dialysis-dependence.

Conclusion. Renal failure in critical illness should be treated aggressively. The increased cost is justified by good survival rates. Although number of OSF, age > 65, and Apache 2 predicted risk of death were good overall indicators of outcome, none could be used to predict outcome.

2

β_2-M Removal in HDF

G. Pratesi, G. Calabrese, A.G. Aleo, G. Vagelli, A. Mazzotta, M. Vanni, M. Gonella

Renal Unit, Laboratory of Clinical Pathology, General Hospital, Casale Monferrato, Italy

The effect of variations of reinfusate volume (RV) and session duration (SD) upon β_2-M removal was studied in HDF using various membranes (M) with high area.

In 5 patients, polyamide 1.6 (PA), AN69 1.6, PMMA 2.1, PAN 110 2.2m^2 were used varying either RV (23 ± 1 vs 11 ± 1 L/session) while keeping SD unchanged (222 ± 26 min), or SD (210 vs 270 min) while keeping RV unchanged (19 ± 2 L/session). In all cases QB was 400, QD 450 ml/min; TMP, and consequently UF, varied according to the HDF schedule and the M employed. The percent plasma β_2-M decrease(Δ sβ_2-M) and the total β_2-M extraction in the ultrafiltrate-dialysate (β_2-M E) were measured at each session. The postdialysis s β_2-M was corrected according to the variation of body weight.

With larger RV, Δsβ_2-M was higher with PMMA (72 ± 2 vs 59 ± 3, $p < 0.01$), AN69 (69 ± 2 vs 59 ± 4, $p < 0.02$), PAN (73 ± 1 vs 67 ± 3, NS) and remained unchanged with PA (70 ± 5 vs 68 ± 3) ; β_2-ME did not change significantly for each M (ranging from 28 for

PMMA to 136 mg for PAN). With longer SD, $\Delta s\beta_2$-M was higher for PMMA (65 ± 8 vs 57 ± 9, $p<0.005$), AN69 (72 ± 4 vs 67 ± 2, $p<0.025$), and remained unchanged for PAN (76 ± 4 vs 74 ± 3) and PA (75 ± 6 vs 76 ± 4) ; β_2-ME did not change significantly for each M (ranging from 37 for PMMA to 445 mg for PAN).

The different β_2-M handling by the employed M, while changing either RV or SD, could be attributed to their dissimilar absorptive capacity. Therefore, in HDF, RV and SD should be adjusted for each M in order to improve β_2-M removal, also taking into account the possible role of the M area.

3

7 Years Experience with The Brachiosubclavian Fistula for Hemodialysis

Siegfried Gutschi, Hubert Hauser

University Klinik für Chirurgie A-8036 Graz, Auenbruggerplatz 29

There is an increasing number of patients for hemodialysis with poor vascular access.

If fistulas with autologuous veins are not available we implant a brachiosubclavian shunt for dialysis.

A PTFE prostheses or biograft is implanted between the distal brachial artery and the subclavian vein in infraclavicular position.

We implanted 130 PTFE grafts and 32 OMNIFLOW prostheses in a 7 years period.

Graft infection was seen in 11 cases only in PTFE grafts. Thrombotic shunt occlusions occurred in both groups. Aneurysms could be observed only as false aneurysms. Only once surgical procedure had to be performed.

In spite of excellent venous outflow stenoses of the venous anastomoses were the limiting factor for graft function.

The cumulative patiency rate was estimated by life table method. The actuarial function rate for all grafts was 75.3% after two years. The function rate only for OMNIFLOW biografts was slightly higher with a percentage of 78.3 in the same period.

These fistulas have an ideal venous outflow. In case of symptoms of venous obstruction early angiography of the fistulas and PTA and stent implantation are recommended.

4

Indications of Chemoprophylaxis for Tuberculosis in Patients with Chronic Renal Failure

Hou Fan-fan, Zhang Xun, Ren Dong-xuan

Department of Nephrology, Nanfang Hospital, Guangzhou 510515 PRC

Mycobacterial infection poses a very important problem in renal transplantation programmes. Chemoprophylaxis for tuberculosis (TB) should be used in selected patients because of a high prevalence of disseminated TB, but the recommendations for prophylaxis are still confusing. In this study, the indications of prophylaxis for TB in these patients were approached. Mycobacterial infections occurred in 39 out of 830 (4.7%) CRF patients, 58.9% (23/39) of them had TB symptoms within 12 months after hemodialysis (HD) or transplantation. Patients with personal history of TB or recent contact with active TB patients had a higher incidence of TB there after than those without such a history (33.3% vs 4.5%, $p<0.05$). Active TB occurred in 27.3% of patients with abnormal chest radiography on admission (i.e., calcification, pleural thickening and hilar prominence), the incidence was 6 times as high as that in patients with negative chest radiograph. 47.4% of patients with positive serum anti-PPD-IgG developed TB after HD or transplantation, but only 2.3% of patients with negative serum anti-PPD-IgG did ($p<0.01$). Tuberculin skin test had little value in identifying these patients at risk, the difference in TB incidence between patients with positive and negative skin test was not statistically significant, also no differences could be found in TB incidence between patients with and without diabetes, rheumatic diseases, hypoalbuminemia, or aged and non-aged patients. We therefore suggest that prophylaxis for TB should be given to patients with one or more of the following: (1) History of TB or contact with active TB patients; (2) Abnormal chest radiography; (3) Positive serum anti-PPD-IgG.

5

Mycobacterial Infection in CRF Patients with or without Renal Replacement Therapy

Zhang Xun, Hou Fan-fan, Wang Wan-mei

Department of Nephrology, Nanfang Hospital, Guangzhou, 510515, PRC

Active mycobacterial infection developed in 40 of 978 CRF patients with or without renal replacement therapy during a five-year period. The incidence was 4.1% and was 10 times higher than that in the general population. The onset of symptoms was within 1 year after dialysis or kidney transplant in 68%. 82.5% of the patients had predominantly extrapulmonary disease and most of these were lymph nodes infection. the diagnosis of mycobacterial infection was still obscured, tuberculin sensitivity was present only in 6.4% of the patients and examination of sputum and other fluid for mycobacteria was usually unrewarding. Detecting serum anti-PPD-IgG level might be a valuable diagnostic method, because 85% of patients with active tuberculosis showed positive results. Measuring serous exudate and urine anti-PPD-IgG level by ELISA or M. tuberculosis DNA by PCR might be helpful in the diagnosis of tuberculosis serositides and urinary tract mycobacterial infection.

6

Effects on RBC Immune in Uremic Patients Treated with Recombinant Human Erythropoietin

Shi Yue-xian, Fan-fan Hou, Xun Zhang, Jian-ping Jiang

Department of Nephrology, Nanfang Hospital, Guangzhou, 510515, PRC

The relationship between the impairment of RBC immune function in uremic patients and the deficiency of EPO production was studied in vivo and vitro. Thirty-five uremic patients with a mean dialysis period 21.4 months were divided into: group A (n = 15, treated with rHu-EPO, mean time was 7.8 months) and group B (n = 20, untreated with rHu-EPO). Nine healthy volunteers were used as controls. Expression of C3b receptors (C3bR) on RBC isolated from peripheral blood were measured by C3bR rosette test. The results showed there was no statistical difference between expression of C3bR on RBC obtain from group A and that from the controls (17.57 ± 8.13 vs 19.33 ± 3.75). Expression of C3bR began to increase two weeks after treatment with rHu-EPO. Positive correlations were found between the expression level of C3bR and the period of rHu-EPO treatment and the increase of Hb ($r = 0.705$ and 0.758, $p < 0.01$). No correlation was found between the expression level of C3bR and the level of Hb and the period of dialysis. Expression of C3bR in group B (10.85 ± 5.75) was significantly lower than that in group A and the controls ($p < 0.01$). RBC from eight patients of group B were incubated with or without rHu-EPO for 72 hours, both of the expression of C3bR were higher than pre-incubation (16.75 ± 5.88, 15.75 ± 3.62 vs 12.54 ± 4.16, $p < 0.01$) but lower than normal ($p <$ 0.05 and 0.01), there was no difference about expression of C3bR on RBC noted between two condition, which indication that rHu-EPO can not improve the expression of RBC directly. These suggest that the immune function of erythrocyte is deficient in uremic patients, and rHu-EPO can improve the function by way of stimulating the production of RBC and increasing the number of erythrocytes.

7

The Level of Endotoxic Antibody in Hemodialysis Patients

Yang Min, Hou Fan-fan, Zhang Xun

Department of Nephrology, Nanfang Hospital, Guangzhou, PRC

Endotoxins are often present in dialysate. They are derived from gram-negative bacteria, expecially Pseudomonas, E. coli and Serratia. It has been thought that they can pass through dialyzer membranes. To investigate this, serum endotoxin antibody level was measured by enzyme-linked immunosorbent assays in maintenance hemodialysis patients. The results showed that the serum level of endotoxin antibody in dialysis patients was significantly higher than that in non-dialysis chronic renal failure patients and normal controls ($p < 0.001$). In the first three months of dialysis, a distinct increase in serum endotoxin antibody level was noted, which was positively correlated with the time of dialysis ($r = 0.254$). The serum endotoxin antibody level was significantly higher in patients using cuprophan membrane dialyzer when compared with those using cellulose acetate membrane dialyzer ($p < 0.05$)

8

Effects of Epidermal Growth Factor (EGF) on Proliferation of Human Peritoneal Mesothelial Cells (HPMC)

Yan Zang, Fan Fan H, Man Qiu Y

Department of Nephrology, Nanfang Hospital. Guangzhou, 510515, PRC

To investigate the expression of epidermal growth factor receptor (EGF-R) on human peritoneal mesothelial cells (HPMC) and the effects of EGF cultured from different time and dosage treatment on the proliferation of HPMC, long-term cultures of peritoneal mesothelial cells from human omentum were established in vitro. The purity of the cell population was assessed by morphologic and immunocytochemical criteria. Five HPMC cultures were analyzed for EGF effect. The results showed that EGF-R existed on the surfaced of HPMC by immunohistochemical staining. The proliferation of HPMC stimulated with EGF was increased significantly ($p < 0.01$) comparing with controls in a does-dependent measured by ^{3}H-thymidine incorporation. There was a maximal stimulating index (SI) at a concentration of 50ng/ml EGF. The results indicate that the effect of EGF on HPMC proliferation may have some significance on the repairment and functional recovery of those injured peritoneum.

9

Protective Effect of Removing LPS, TNF, IL-1 from Circulation on The Experimental Endotoxic Shock Lung

Zhang Guo-hua, Hou Fan-fan Zhang Xun

Department of Nephrology, Nan Fang Hospital, Guangzhou, 510515, PRC

Hemoperfusion with activated charcoal (Ⅱ group) or amberlite XAD-7 (Ⅲ group) significantly decreased the circulated LPS, IL-1 or TNF levels in the early stage of experimental model of endotoxic shock in rats. After 2 hours of hemoperfusion, the blood WBC counts of two treated groups were $4.0 \pm 0.4 \times 10^9$/L, $3.9 \pm 0.4 \times 10^9$/L respectively, which were significantly higher than that in sham group (Ⅰ group) ($3.1 \pm 0.2 \times 10^9$/L, $p < 0.01$ in all). Both the WBC count in bronchoalveolar lavage fluid and pulmonary coefficient were significantly lower than that in Ⅰ group ($p < 0.01$ in all) when compared with the Ⅰ group. The pathological lessions were ameliorative and less infiltrating neutrophils were noted (29.6 ± 7.9/rlp. 34.5 ± 4.1/rlp vs 48.6 ± 6.6/HP, $p < 0.05$ in all). It suggested that removal of deleterious mediators from circulation by hemoperfusion may be of protective effect on endotoxic shock lung.

10

Beta-2-Microglobulin (β_2-M) Kinetics during Hemodialysis (HD) with Different Membranes

Stetsyuk E., Siniukhin V., Plemiashov G

Institute of Urology, Moscow, Russia

There are not enough data on β_2-M kinetics during HD comparing different membranes in the same patients The aim of this study was to investigate if blood membrane interactions influence the level of β_2-M during HD with polysulfon low flux F6 (Fresenius) and cellulose acetate-N Altra Nova-170 (Althin) hollow fiber dialyzers. 6 patients entered this study. All patients were treated with maintance HD. Blood samples were taken immediately before HD and after 15, 90 and 210 min from HD start. β_2-M concentrations were measured by

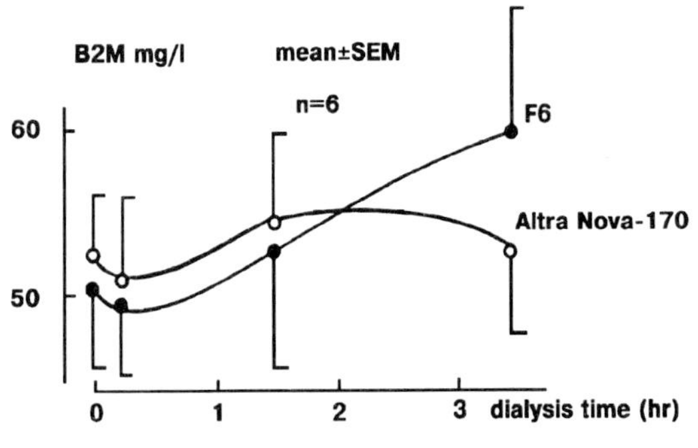

Microparticle Enzyme Immunoassay (Abbott). The results expressed as mean ± SEM (mg/l).

During HD with F6 β_2-M level at 210 min was significantly higher than before HD (Wilcoxon test $p < 0.05$). There was no significant change of β_2-M during HD with Altra Nova-170. Ultrafiltration rate was the same in both series. In some patients we observed the phenomenon of acute β_2-M decrease after HD start. The phenomenon looked like well-known leucopenic effect and may be connected with cells activation. We think that polysulfon low flux activates β_2-M generation during HD.

11

The Prophylactic Effect of Long-Term $CaCO_3$ Treatment on Aluminum Osteopathy

X. Zhang, F. F. Hou

Department of Nephrology, Nanfang Hospital, Guangzhou, PRC

Aluminum (Al) -related osteopathy has been identified in dialysis patients receiving phosphate (P) binder containing Al. In this study, 30 uremia patients were treated with $CaCO_3$ as P binder when they were first diagnosed and continued to at least 24 months. The doses were adjusted aiming at a serum P level < 2mmol/L. 25 patients who had been receiving Al $(OH)_3$ for the same duration were selected as controls. The results showed that serum P were well controlled in patients given $CaCO_3$. No difference could be seen in mean levels of serum calcium, alkaline phosphatases and parathyroid hormone between patients treated with $CaCO_3$ and with Al $(OH)_3$. However, the mean serum aluminum level in the group treated with $CaCO_3$ was significantly lower. Bone histology showed that aluminum deposition could be seen in 52% (13/25) of patients treated with Al $(OH)_3$, 12 of whom presented low-turnover or mixed renal osteodystrophy. However, only 10% (3/30) of patients treated with $CaCO_3$ exhibited aluminum deposition in bone ($p < 0.01$). These data indicate that $CaCO_3$ is an effective Al free P binder. Its ling-term administration may stop the progression of aluminum osteopathy developed with Al intake.

12

Change of Lymphocyte Secretion Function in Hemodialysis Patients

Shi Yue-xian, Hou Fan-fan, Zhang Xun

Department of Nephrology, Nan Fang Hospital, Guangzhou, PRC

Some secretion function of lymphocyte usually changed markerly in end-stage renal disease patients maintained on long-term hemodialysis (HD). The secretion of β_2-microglobulin (β_2-M), IgG, IgA and IgM by lymphocyte, and the effect of different dialysis membranes on which is studied in vitro. Lymphocytes were isolated from three long-term HD patients and three healthy controls. Cells were cultured with Cuprophan, Hemophan, Polyacrylonitrile (PAN), Polysulfone (PS), Polyacryl and Cellulose Acetate membranes as well as blank respectively. β_2-M, IgG, IgA and IgM concentrations in the supernatants were measured after 72 hours of culture by RIA and ELISA techniques. β_2-M release from lymphocytes obtain from HD patients was significantly more than that from healthy subjects (214.5 ± 3.7 vs 160.4 ± 12.4, $p < 0.05$). Under the presence of PAN or PS membranes, the concentrations of β_2-M was less than that of control in both group (127.3 ± 21.2, 132.8 ± 9.1 vs 160.4 ± 12.4; 161.6 ± 29.5, 169.5 ± 8.3 vs 214.5 ± 30.7, $p < 0.05$), even the absorptive capacitys of those membranes were taken into account. IgG, IgA concentrations in patients group were significantly lower than those in healthy group (251.8 ± 9.5 vs 326.4 ± 33.6; 38.7 ± 17.2 vs 111.4 ± 23.7, $p < 0.05$), and no significant difference of IgM concentrations was found between two groups. All Immune-globulin concentrations studied remained unchanged under six membranes presence. The result showed that the increase of β_2-M release from lymphocyte may be one of the causes of accumulation of circulating β_2-M in long-term HD patients, and dialysis membrane have no stimulation effect on its secretion, on the contrary, some could suppress it. The capacities of lymphocyte to secrete IgG, IgA in uremic patients were significantly lower than those in healthy subjects, which may be among the factors of immune deficiency in uremic patients.

13

Effects of Interleukin-1 (IL-1) on Secretion of Extracellular Matrix by Human Peritoneal Mesothelial Cells (HPMC)

Yan Zang, Zhi Qing Liu, Fan Fan Hou

Department of Nephrology, Nanfang Hospital. Guangzhou, PRC

Peritoneal ultrafitration failure, which resulted from extensive peritoneal fibrosis caused by bacterial infection, was the main cause to drop-out CAPD for most patients. Mononuclear phagocytic cells, as a first barrier during defence bacterial infection, were increased and produced a amount of IL-1 in peritonitis. In order to study the relationship between IL-1 and peritoneal fibrosis, HPMC was separated and cultured with different concentration of IL-1 for 72 hours in vitro. The effects of IL-1 on secretion of extracellular matrix by HPMC was observed to detect the roles of IL-1 in the process of peritoneal fibrosis by measuring the content of fibronectin (FN) and IV-type collagen with ELISA method. The results showed that high concentration of IL-1 (50ng/ml) can stimulate HPMC producing extracellular matrix, and the contents of FN and IV-type collagen in supernatant were increased obviously ($p < 0.01$) compairing with controls. The results indicate that it may be one of the main causes of peritoneal fibrosis that HPMC produced extracellular matrix stimulated by IL-1.

14

Application of Back-Infused Peritoneal Fluid in the Treatment of Hemodialysis Associated Ascites

Ji Dan, Lin Zhen, Yang Tiechen

Department of Nephrology, Nanfang Hospital, Guangzhou, 510515, PRC

The hemodialysis patients are often accompanied with intractable peritoneal fluid and it is not effective to treat with the ordinary method, such as restricted water and salt, given diuretic for the patients. Infusion of plasma albumin is still expensive and risk of viral infections. The more peritoneal fluid is extracted, the more protein from peritoneal fluid is lost and in the meantime, decreased plasma colloid osmotic pressure will be got more peritoneal fluid accumulated in the peritoneal cavity. Back-infused peritoneal fluid can be avoided of mentioned disadvantage. As the extracted peritoneal fluid passes through a high flux filter excess water and solute can be removed and concentrated fluid can be given by blood line into the patients. We have treated 12 cases (male 9, female 3) of HD patients with intractable peritoneal fluid in the 34 times treatments and got good results.

Back-infused peritoneal fluid method: Fix high-flux filter on the hemodialysis machine, linking Arterio-Venous (A-V) vascular access. Inserting puncture tubing into the rectovesical pouch under the strictly aseptic manipulation. Collecting peritoneal fluid into the sterile bottle (contain 5 mg heparin), which passes through filter, excess water and solute can be removed from peritoneal fluid and the concentrated peritoneal fluid can be infused by vascular access.

The important points in the treatment are as follows: (1) Measure the blood pressure, pulse rate, and respiratory rate and check peritoneal fluid routine examination and blood biochemical examination before treatment. (2) The treatment is performed by strictly aseptic manipulation and keep the tubes, peritoneal fluid and reagents in the aseptic condition. (3) Monitor the vital signs, peritoneal fluid condition, observe closely the working condition of machine and its various tubes during the treatment. (4) Prevent bleeding, infection, hypertension and heart failure, control of fluid input, high vitamin and high nutrition diet should be given after the treatment.

15

Endotoxins Elimination by Xenospleen in Peritonitis

Sh. Kasimov, B. Kasimov

Research Centre of Surgery of Ministry of Health, Tashkent, Republic of Uzbekistan

For elimination and withdrawing of endotoxins a pig spleen was used. In 73 patients in toxic phase of peritonitis hemoperfusion via xenospleen (XS) operation of biohemosorption (BHS) was performed.

BHS was made on extracorporeal contour with the use of "Unitrol 05" hemoprocessor. BHS effectiveness was evaluated at the generally clinical signs, hemodynamics, hepatic and renal function, blood counts, leukocytic index of intoxication (LII), toxins level of mean molecular mass (TMM), serotonin and histamine and also morphologic picture of XS and erythrocytes of patients.

In the result of observations it was established that after BHS operations the patients state, hemodynamics improved, the leukocytes number reduced by 38%, neutrophiles with toxic dependence by 31.5% TMM by 49.5, LII by 58.3%, serotonin and histamine by 46.5%. Index of glomerular filtration increased by 62.8%. In morphologic picture of XS the increase of red pulp and dilatation of blood vessels and echocytic and stomatocytic alterated erythrocytes accumulation in sinusoid lumen were revealed.

Thus, BHS was the effective method of elimination and withdrawing of endotoxins from patients organism with severe forms of toxemia.

16

Host Responses to Hepatitis B Virus Infection in Dialysis Patients

Hi Bahl Lee

Hyonam Kidney Laboratory, Soon Chun Hyang University, Seoul, Korea

Uremia is associated with impaired immune responses and dialysis patients display altered immune responses to hepatitis B virus (HBV) infection. The incidence of HBV infection is abnormally high among dialysis patients and the HBV antigenemia persists for a long period in these patients. Dialysis patients have lower rate of antibody response to hepatitis B vaccine and lower anti-HBs titer in those who respond.

We found that T cells from dialysis patients who did not respond to vaccine had decreased in vitro proliferative response to anti-CD_3 mAb but normal response to combination of anti-CD_2mAb, 9-1 and 9.6, suggesting functional defects of monocyte as well as T cell. T cells from uremic carriers of HbsAg had significantly decreased release of 2'5'-oligoadenylate synthetase in response to PHA, suggesting defective production of γ-interferon (IFN). Peripheral blood mononuclear cells (PBMC) from uremic carriers produced normal amount of IgG in response to PWM or combination of PWM and γ-IFN but not anti-HBs in response to PWM alone, HBsAg alone, or to combinations of PWM and HBsAg, PWM and γ-IFN, or HBsAg and γ-IFN.

When purified B cells from uremic carrier were cultured with T cells and/or monocytes from healthy responder to vaccine and stimulated with PWM there was a significant increase in anti-HBs and the response was even greater when the cells were stimulated with combination of PWM and γ-IFN.

These results suggest that uremic carrier B cells have the potential to produce anti-HBs in the presence of normal T cells and monocytes.

17

New Surface Treated Catheters for Blood Access for Extracorporeal Detoxification Methods

R. Bambauer, P. Mestres, R. Schiel, P. Sioshansi

University of Saarland, Homburg/Saar, FRG Spire Corporation, Bedford, Mass, USA

Infection, thrombosis and stenosis are among the most common complications of blood-contacting catheters and are caused by surface properties of the catheter materials. Ion beam-based processes such as ion implantation and ion beam-assisted de- position affect only the outer micron of the treated surface. These processes were therefore used on common catheter materials.

The surface treated process uses ion implantation to improve the surface properties of silicone rubber with a high degree of reproducibility while bulk properties such as tensile strength, bulk modulus, flexibility etc. are maintained. The catheter with silver treated surfaces, ion beam assisted deposition was used to create an infection resistant "actively sterile" coating. This coating is bacteriocidal on contact, minimally leading in the body biocompatible etc.

Large bore catheters for blood access in hemodialysis without and with treated surface with silver or silicone (Spi-Silicone, Spi Argent I and II) were investigated after removal with a scanning electron microscope and for bacterial colonization.

In 42 large bore catheters (in situ time x = 21.3 days) of 3 different materials deposits of fibrin, protein and blood cells on the inner and outer surface were seen. This second layer covered the entire surface after 3 days and increased to a thickness of 3 to 90 μm during the following days. Bacterial colonisation was observed in 38.1%. In contrast to these results the 67 catheters with the treated outer surface (Spi silicone n = 28, in situ time x = 24.1 days: Spi-Argent I n = 22, x = 27.0 days, Spi-Argent II n-17, x = 28.5 days) showed a very low thrombogenecity and in regard of the in situ time, if at all, only small deposits. The infection rate was with 8.9% significant lower than in the untreated from 1.4 to 2.8 μ/l after the average in situ time of 27.0 days. Some days later normalization of the silver concentration was reached. These surface treatment processes can be readily applied to blood contacting catheters to make them thrombus and infection resistant.

18

LDL-Apheresis versus Lipid-Lowering Drugs in Treatment of Severe Hypercholesterolemia

R. Schiel[a], R. Bambauer[b], U.A. Müller[a]

[a]University of Jena, Medical School, Jena
[b]University of Saarland, Homburg, Germany

High lipoprotein concentrations seems to be strongly, in a dose dependent manner, to an increased incidence of atherosclerosis. A total of 47 patients suffering from severe hypercholesterolemia were matched to treatment with LDL-apheresis (BAXTER[R], KANEKA[R], LIPOPAK[R], 24 patients, aged 49.5 ± 11.5 vs, BMT 26.6 ± 3.1 kg/m^2).

After treatment periods of 44.4 ± 14.3 (apheresis group, n-2055 treatment sessions) and 33.5 ± 15.9 (drug group) months, respectively, the ensuing results revealed significant differences ($p < 0.0001$) :

-47.1% vs 12.5% for total cholesterol, -47.2% vs -21.4% for LDL, +8.5% vs +9.0% for HDL, -52.1 -% vs -13.3% for LDL/HDL-ratio, -36.0% vs -16.3% for triglycerides and -26.6% vs +1.4% for Lp (a). With LDL-apheresis the fibrinogen concentration was reduced by 14.3%. In the apheresis group one patient died from myocardial infarction vs non fatal myocardial infarction and the manifestation of coronary heart disease in three cases in the drug group. There were no serious side effects in both groups. All patients out of the apheresis group experienced an increase in clinical performance. But, psychological wellbeing (assessed according to BRADLEY et al.) of these patients was lower than that of the drug group (42.3 ± 8.9 vs 50.2 ± 9.9 points, $p < 0.002$).

Often the former being more depressive, anxious and have less energy. The present long-term results show that the efficacy of lipid-lowering very favourably influences the clinical performance and prognosis psychological wellbeing. In respect of clinical and laboratory results, LDL-apheresis seems a safe and the most effective therapy.

19

LDL-Apheresis in The Treatment of Familial Hypercholesterolemia-Six Years Experience

R. Bambauer, R. Schiel, H.E. Keller, R. Latza

University of Saarland, Homburg, Germany

Familial hypercholesterolemia (FH) is a genetic disease characterized by an overabundance of cholesterol carrying low density lipoprotein (LDL) in the blood. LDL is considered to be one of the major risk factors for atherosclerosis and coronary heart disease (CHD). In total 30 patients (13 males, 17 females, aged 44.2 ± 14.8, 21-67 ys) with FH (2 with homozygous, 28 with heterozygous), resistant to diet and lipid-lowering drugs, were treated since 1989 (42.6 ± 18.9, 2-81 months) with LDL-apheresis (BAXTER[R], KANEKA[R], LIPOPAK[R]). Prior to LDL apheresis 23/30 patiens suffered from CHD. 5/23 patients had suffered 9 myocardial infarctions. Initially 20/23 patients suffered intermittently from symptoms of angina, exertional dyspnoea and claudication.

Following 2561 treatment sessions (22.1 ± 3.4 sessions per year and patient, perfusion volume 5371 ± 1749ml) lipid concentrations were reduced significantly ($p < 0.001$). In particular, in respect of Lp (a), LDL, but also in respect of total cholesterol and triglycerides,

Table to Abstract 19

	Trig	Chol	LDL	HDL	LpA	ApoB	Fibr
Pre apher	501	407	289	41	28	273	472
after 1 y	305	229	158	43	18	192	378
after 3 y	289	203	141	46	21	164	364
at the end	302	215	148	45	21	167	351

Mean values (mg/dl) under aphersis

the different methods revealed different degrees of efficacy.

Severs side effects such as shock symptoms or allergic reactions were very rare (0.4). In the course of treatment with LDL-apheresis an improvement in general well-being and increased performance was experienced by 29/30 patients. No further cardiac complaints were documented. A reduction of nitrate medication was observed in 17/23 patients. Regular treatment with LDL-apheresis seems to be able to prevent and to stabilize progressive CHD in patients suffering from FH.

....

20

LDL-Apheresis in Two Patients with Extremely Elevated Lipoprotein (A)

R. Bambauer, R. Schiel, R. Latza

University of Saarland, Homburg, Germany

Hyperlipidemia and elevated lipoprotein (a) (Lp (a)) levels are associated with increased risk for atherosclerosis and coronary heart disease (CHD). Two caucasian males suffering from heterozygous familial hypercholesterolemia and extremely elevated Lp (a) levels, resistant to diet and lipid lowering drugs, and no other risk factors were treated with LDL-apheresis. Two different methods were used: One patient, aged 42 ys was treated for 55 months with dextran-sulfate adsorption (KANEKA^R, Japan). The second, 36 ys old patient was treated for 15 months with an immunoadsorption system (special Lp (a) columns, LIPOPAKR, Russia). Following a total of 154 LDL-apheresis, respectively, the ensuing results revealed substantial differences. Using the immunoadsorption system with special columns containing antibodies against Lp (a), a significant reduction ($p < 0.001$) of Lp (a) of 57% vs 43% with dextran-sulfate adsorption could be reached. Total cholesterol dropped by 24.9% vs 29.6%. LDL by 35.0% vs 48.5%, triglyceride by 41.3% vs 45.2%, fibrinogen by 13.1% vs 18.2% and HDL increase by 3.8% vs 4.2% ($p < 0.001$). Pretreatment both patients suffered three myocardial infarctions. Four and six coronary angiographies with two and four percutaneous transluminal angioplasties (PTCA) were necessary. Since treatment with LDL-apheresis neither myocardial infarctions nor cardiac complaints were observed. Both patients experienced an improvement in general well-being and increased performance. Available data suggest that lipid-lowering, in particular lowering of extremely elevated Lp (a) levels, favourably influences the clinical performance and prognosis of patients with CHD. Up to now, LDL-apheresis and in particular immunoadsorption with special Lp (a) columns seems to be the sures and most effective therapy for reduction of elevated Lp (a) levels.

....

21

Design of Nonthrombogenic Polymer Surfaces for Blood Contacting Medical Devices

Sung Wan Kim

Department of Pharmaceutics and Pharmaceutical Chemistry, Center for Controlled Chemical Delivery, Biomedical Polymers Research Building, #205, University of Utah, Salt Lake City, Utah 84112

Although significant progress has been made in the design of blood compatible polymers for the past decades, there is no ideal polymer surface which is comparable with a natural endothelial surface in preventing surface induced thrombosis and maintaining hemostasis. This is due to the complex pattern of protein and cellular interactions with foreign surfaces, which still demands defining a proven hypothesis to develop non-thrombogenic surfaces. Synthesis of new polymers with optimal mechanical properties and the in vitro and in vivo characterization of these surfaces will require many more years work.

In this presentation, the surface modification of existing medical polymers for the improvement of blood compatibility will be introduced. Surface immobilizing of heparin onto polyurethane, coatings of polyurethane-PEO-heparin graft copolymer, and a coating of thermosensitive polymers on polyurethane will be discussed. In addition, the design of an endothelial cell/polymer matrix and new concepts involving gene therapy for transfection of smooth muscle cells will be discussed. The biological response of these designed systems in vitro, ex vivo and in vivo should provide state of the art materials for the specific application of controlling thrombosis and solving biocompatibility problems.

22

Photochemical Surface Process Technologies for Advanced Artificial Organs

Takehisa Matsuda

Department of Bioengineering, National Cardiovascular Center Research Insititute 5-7-1 Fujishirodai, Suita, Osaka 565, Japan

The reliability of advanced, functional artificial organs largely depends on biocompatible surface design. In this talk, novel surface process technologies providing desired biocompatibility such as blood- or tissue-compatibility at a given portion of fabricated device with micron-order dimensional precision. The principle behind is to utilize photochemistries enabling covalent bonding of adsorbants to substrate surfaces. Our photochemically-driven surface processing created functional surfaces, which cover a wide spectrum of surface properties from very hydrophilic to very hydrophobic surfaces and from albuminated to heparinized surfaces. Cell-adhesive or non-adhesive surface design can be easily realized using these techniques. Photo-induced surface process technologies may promise to upgrade biocompatibility of complex-shaped devices.

23

Protein Losses in Continuous Venovenous Hemofiltration and Hemodialysis (CVVH & CVVHD)

Michele H. Mokrzycki[a], *Andre A. Kaplan*[b]

[a]Albert Einstein College of Medicine & Bronx Municipal Hospital Center, Bronx NY

[b]University of Connecticut Health Center, Farmington CT, USA

Continuous hemofiltration has become an increasingly popular means of renal replacement therapy in the severely ill ICU patient. As a possible disadvantage to this therapy, hemofiltrate (HF) protein losses have been reported to be high when analyzed by the Lowry and Biuret methods, yielding values of 1.3 g/L and 0.8 g/L, respectively: equivalent to total losses of 20 to 40 gms of protein/day. Based on published sieving characteristics, one would anticipate low HF protein losses with solute clearance limited to a maximum of 20 to 30,000 daltons. Thus, the previously reported levels of protein losses may be an overestimate resulting from the use of relatively inaccurate methodology.

We evaluated HF protein losses using a highly sensitive microprotein reagent method (pyrogallol red). Filtrate was obtained from 4 CVVH treatments and 2 CVVHD treatments. Amicon 20 diafilters (2 CVVH and 1 CVVHD) and Fresenius HF-80 filters (2 CVVH and 1 CVVHD) were tested. For the Amicon filters, mean HF protein concentration was 0.034 g/L (range 0.01-0.05 g/L, n = 9, mean serum protein 35 g/L). For the Fresenius hemofilters mean protein concentration was 0.085 g/L (range 0.03 to 0.10 g/L, n = 4, serum protein 69 g/L). Despite large daily HF/Dialysate volumes of up to 45 liters/day, total daily protein losses were 4.5 g or less.

We conclude that, when analyzed by an appropriately accurate methodology, protein losses during large volume CVVH or CVVHD are substantially less than previously reported.

24

Effects of Recombinant Human Erythropoietin (r-HuEPO) on Nutritional Status in Continuous Ambulatory Peritoneal Dialysis (CAPD) Patients

SB Kim, JY Kang, S Park, DH Moon, JS Park, CD Hong

Asan Medical Center, University of Ulsan, Seoul, Korea

Effects of r-HuEPO on nutritional status were studied longitudinally in 9 CAPD patients. Patients with hemoglobin less than 8g/dL were enrolled. Their age ranged 38 to 70 (median 48) and underlying disease was diabetes mellitus in 6 patients. r-HuEPO was given subcutaneously thrice weekly to achieve a hemoglobin concentration of 10g/dL, then had been adjusted to maintain 10-11g/dL. Following variables were measured in baseline, and at 3 and 6 months of treatment: Body mass index (BMI), triceps skin fold (TSF), midarm muscle area (MAMA), albumin, prealbumin, transferrin, insulin like growth factor-1 (IGF-1), muscle mass of lower extremities by dual photon absorptiometry, Kt/V and normalized protein catabolic rate (nPCR). The results are as follows (mean ± S.D.) :

Table to Abstract 24

	Baseline	3 months	6 months
BMI (Kg/m^2)	21.6±1.8	22.5±1.7	24.3±0.9
TSF (mm)	11.8±5.0	13.0±5.7	12.8±3.4
MAMA (cm^2)	25.4±4.9	28.3±6.1	28.3±6.7
Albumin (g/dl)	3.5±0.4	3.6±0.4	3.7±0.7
Prealbumin (mg/dl)	29.4±8.1	37.9±5.8*	40.7±9.0*
Transferrin (mg/dl)	158±37	213±61*	202±39*
IGF-1 (ng/ml)	332±139	316±53	415±206
Muscle mass (Kg)	14.5±2.7	13.7±2.6	14.4±1.8
Kt/V	2.1±0.6	1.9±0.4	1.9±0.2
nPCR (g/Kg/d)	1.1±0.4	1.0±0.1	0.9±0.1

* $p < 0.05$ when compared with baseline

Conclusion. Prealbumin and transferrin known as early nutritional indicator increased after r-HuEPO administration in CAPD patients. The effects of r-HuEPO on other nutritional indices need longer follow-up.

25

Bacterial Proliferation in Peritoneal Dialysis Effluent after Exposure to Acidic Dialysis Solution: Implications for Neutral pH Formulations

Holmes CJ, Hickey G, Cipolla P, Kubey W

Renal and Applied Science Divisions, Baxter Healthcare, McGaw Park and Round Lake, IL

Numerous *in vitro* studies have reported that short exposure of mesothelial cells and leukocytes to acidic lactate-based peritoneal dialysis solutions (PDS) significantly impairs their function. However, as the susceptibility to peritonitis in PD patients must be the balance between host defense and bacteria to acidic PDS on their subsequent ability to survive and proliferate in dialysate was studied.

Overnight cultures of *S. aureus* ATCC 25923 and *P. aeruginosa* ATCC 27853 were harvested, washed twice and resuspended in normal saline to a concentration of 106 cfu/ml. Then 100 μl of each suspension was individually inoculated into 9.9 ml of lactate-based PDS at pH 5.2, 5.5, 5.8 and 7.4 and phosphate buffered saline. The pH of the PDS was adjusted as needed with $NaHCO_3$. After shaking for 15 minutes at 37℃ in closed containers, 1.5 ml was inoculated into 13.5 ml of pooled human dialysis effluent and proliferation quantitated at 37℃ over 24 hours.

Control studies showed that the selected strains of *S. aureus* and *P. aeruginosa* increased by 3.0 log_{10} and 3.8 log_{10} in effluent over 24 hours respectively. Pre-exposure of bacteria to any of the test fluids, including those at pH 5.2, did not affect their subsequent proliferation in effluent and growth curves were superimposable. It is concluded that transient exposure of bacteria to acidic lactate-based PDS is unlikely to affect their viability or proliferation in the *in vivo* situation.

26

Bioactive Polymers for the Removal of Blood Cholesterol

Adriaan Bantjes

Department of Chem. Technology, University of Twente, P.O. Box 217, 7500 AE Enschede, The Netherlands

The lipoprotein metabolism and the most important deviations thereof will be discussed in case of familial hypercholesteremia. General treatments of patients with moderately increased LDL levels include dietary and pharmaceutical treatments with a.o. Probucol, Cholestyramine, Compactin and Nicotinic acid. For homozygote and the severe heterozygote familial hypercholesteremia patients extracorporeal blood or plasma treatment is required to lower Low Density Lipoprotein cholesterol levels. In this way severe cardiovascular damage and LDL atherosclerosis can be prevented. Various specific sorbents have been developed for LDL binding a.o. dextrane sulfate/cellulose, microporous cellulose, polyacrylates, chitosan, and the crosslinked sulfated polyvinylalcohol gels we have developed, which will be discussed in detail. This gel type can bind 250 μmol. per ml. gel. The highly atherogenic Lp (a) is also effectively removed, while HDL is not bound.

Other systems for the removal of LDL are based on the precipitation with heparin, hydrolysis by means of immobilized phospholipase A2, and immunosorption by means of immobilized antibodies directed against the LDL apo-B protein mantle. The various apheresis techniques will be discussed as well as their advantages and disadvantages, such as their interaction with blood clotting factors.

Literature: (1) N.Maaskant, A.Bantjes, H.J.M. Kempen, Atherosclerosis, 1986, 62 (2), 159-66 (2) N.Maaskant, A.Bantjes, H.J.M. Kempen, Dev. Hematol. Immunol., 1986, 14, 317-26 (3) Maaskant, Sulfated polyvinylalcohol based low density lipoprotein binders. Report 1986, order No PB-87-208120, 193 pp.

27

Tissue Engineering of a Kidney: Application of Cell and Gene Therapies

H. David Humes

University of Michigan Medical Center and VA Medical Center, Ann Arbor, Michigan, USA

Long-term ex vivo therapy for kidney failure has been achieved. Accordingly, the kidney may be the first solid organ in which tissue engineering constructs can produce an implantable device for long-term in vivo replacement function. To fully replace renal function, a bioartificial kidney requires both a device to maintain blood ultrafiltration performed by glomeruli and a device to substitute transport and regulatory functions of renal tubules. Early prototypes have been developed to reproduce these two functions. Using a single hollow fiber bioreactor, hollow fibers were prelined with various extracellular matrix compounds and seeded with mammalian renal tubule or endothelial cells. After 5-7 days in the bioreactor, confluent growth of cell monolayers was achieved along the inner aspect of the hollow fiber by both morphologic and functional criteria. Permselective convective fluid transfer under physiologic pressure and flow conditions occurred in the filter. To further improve hemocompatibility of the filter, retroviral gene transfer of the thrombin inhibitor, hirudin. into endothelial cells has been accomplished. Transport along transmural hydraulic, osmotic and oncotic pressure differences has also been accomplished in the bioartificial tubule. Thus, early tissue engineered prototypes have been developed to replicate the important physiologic functions of the kidney.

28

Biocompatibility and Dialysis: The Influence of Membrane Characteristics and Heparin on Coagulation and Fibrinolysis

Kreisl J[a], Forster P[b], Schmidt C[c], Deppisch R[c], Fürst P[b], Schneider H[a]

[a]Nephrology and Dialysis Center Stuttgart
[b]Institute of Nutrition and Biological Chemistry, University Hohenheim
[c]Gambro R & D Hechingen, FRG

There is growing evidence that longterm complications in ESRD patients might be attributable to bioincompatibility of extracorporeal blood purification techniques. Stimulation of plasmatic and cellular effector systems, i.e. endothelial cells, fibrinolysis, kallikrein-kinin, coagulation and complement system, are proposed. The potential role of different activation pathways is investigated in a prospective study over a period of 12 months in 24 ESRD-patients. The patients were treated in four periods (3 months each) according to the following protocol; P1: low flux hemodialysis (HD) using cuprophan membranes (CM) ; P2: high flux HD using polyamide membranes (PAM) ; P3: high flux HD using PAM with reduced heparin doses; P4: low flux HD using CM (equivalent to period P1). At the end of each period arterial blood was obtained at the beginning ($t = 0$), after 15 min and at the end of treatment ($t = 240$). Plasma thrombin-antithrombin III (TAT), plasmin-antiplasmin (PAP) and factor XIIa were analysed (ELISA) as indicators of thrombin generation, fibrinolysis and ongoing contact phase activation, respectively. Terminal complement complex (TCC) was measured (ELISA) at $t = 0$ and $t = 15$ min.

TAT concentration at the end of treatment was not significantly changed(P2: 24.6 ± 5.3 vs P3: 20.9 ± 4.9 ug/l), despite reduction in heparin total dose from 6600 (P2) to 4800 IU (P3). In the low heparin period (P3) PAP concentration at $t = 240$ min was lower than in P2 (811 vs 658 ug/l, $p < 0.05$) suggesting diminished endothelial cell derived plasminogen cleavage. Interestingly, this effect was reversed (846 ug/l, $p < 0.05$) when heparin dose was increased in P4. TCC generation was low during treatment with PAM, irrespective of heparin, and high with CM, but remained at a 20% lower level in P4 than in P1. Factor XIIa concentrations could be measured before dialysis in P1 and P3, showing a reduced intrinsic coagulation activity (14.0 vs. 11.4 ng/ml, $p < 0.05$).

Conclusions. Endothelial cell dependent fibrinolysis activity (PAP) is apparently regulated by heparin availability but not by membrane characteristics. Obviously, high-flux dialysis with PAM is associated with lower complement turnover (TCC) and reduced intrinsic coagulation activity (factor XIIa) and enables reduction of heparin dose without increasing thrombin generation (TAT).

It is tempting to speculate that high-flux dialysis with highly biocompatible membranes limits procoagulatory and immunomodulatory activities and thus may beneficially influence the process of arteriosclerosis in ESRD patients.

29

The Control of Protein Metabolism in uremia

George A. Kaysen

University of California Davis, and the Department of Veteran's Affairs Northern California System of Clinics. Davis and Pleasant Hill CA USA

Many metabolic consequences of renal failure are a result of the inability to normally excrete metabolites or of reduced synthesis of substances produced by the kidney. Low molecular weight peptides such as β_2 microglobulin, normally filtered and catabolized in the proximal tubule accumulate in plasma and may have deleterious effects. Changes in muscle protein metabolism are a consequence of failed proton excretion. The resulting metabolic acidosis causes increased catabolism of proteins in skeletal muscle through activation of the ATP-ubiquitin-proteasome dependent proteolytic pathway. The process is a consequence of acidosis induced augmentation of muscle ubiquitin gene expression and requires the presence of glucocorticoids. Increased proteolysis is followed by oxidation of branch chain essential amino acids. Nitrogen released is transported to liver for hepatic glutamine synthesis. In the absence of renal failure glutamine is transported to the kidney, deaminated, and the ammonia excreted in urine, correcting metabolic acidosis. This cycle is subverted when kidneys are absent. Hepatic secretion of insulin like-growth factor-1 (IGF-I) in response to growth hormone is also reduced. While this may in part be secondary to nutritional changes, renal failure may contribute to hepatic growth hormone unresponsiveness. Decreased IGF-I may lead to growth retardation, adding to the effects of acidosis. Muscle also shows insulin resistance in renal failure. Renal production of both erythropoietin and 1.25 dihydroxycholecalciferol is reduced leading to decreased erthrocyte production and increased transcription of the gene encoding PTH respectively. Both quantitative and qualitative defects also occur in secretion of proteins by a variety of other tissues as well, although the cause of these changes is unknown. Hepatic synthesis of some proteins, such as apolipoprotein A-I is decreased, causing changes in blood lipid levels and metabolism. Albumin synthesis, in contrast is not grossly affected by renal failure, although efficiency of translation may be reduced. Pancreatic protein synthesis and secretion is reduced in uremia, but these changes are of uncertain clinical importance.

30

Study of rHuEPO-Derived Hypertension in Uremic Patients

S. Nakamura[a], K. Kato[a], T. Mitsuma[a], K. Adachi[a], M. Kayama[a], H. Ohashi[b]

[a]Aichi Medical University

[b]Gifu Prefectural Hospital

Introduction. rHuEPO (EPO) is very effective for renal anemia, however, it is noticed to cause hypertension in quite a few patients treated by EPO. The etiology of hypertension is controversial.

Purpose. The aim of this study is to elucidate the cause of hypertension in patients with chronic renal failure (CRF) given EPO.

Methods. Undialyzed patients with CRF (N = 10) and dialyzed patients (N = 15) were selected at random. EPO was discontinued 7 days prior to study. Anti hypertensive agents were also discontinued on the study morning. One hour after supine position, the study was begun with measuring blood pressure (BP) and drawing blood samples for chemical assays such as circulating blood cells, cathecholamines, endothelin-1 (ET-1) and so on

Table to Abstract 30

	RBC (10^4/ml)	Hgb (g/dl)	Hct (%)	ET-1 (pg/ml)	SBP	DBP	MBP	NA (pg/ml)	A (pg/ml)
3000U									
pre	277.4	8.7	26.3	17.3	141.5	98.4	98.4	585.5	26.5
60min	280.0	8.8	26.6	17.5	153.5*	80.0	100.6	478.5	26.0
6000U									
pre	368.0	12.0	36.6	16.4	140.8	70.6	94	442.7	28.5
60min	362.4	11.9	36.4	17.2	153.6*	81.6*	105.6*	415.6	38.9

* $p < 0.05$

EPO was intravenously given 3000U to dialyzed patients and 6000U to undialyzed patients. ET-1 was assayed using extraction method and RIA (normal range: 10.7 ± 0.73 pg/ml: M ± SE).

Results. Results are shown in the table.

Conclusion. Since elevation in BP was detected despite of any increment of RBC and Hct, EPO itself or an unknown factor seem to induce hypertension. The role of ET-1 in hypertension as a cause remains uncertain, although ET-1 increased in some cases.

31

Treatment of Pulmonary Allograft Rejection by Extracorporeal Photo-Chemotherapy (ECP) : A Pilot Study

D.P. Besnier[a], *D. Chabannes*[b], *A. Haloun*[c], *Ph. Despins*[c], *J-L. Michaud*[c], *S. Martin*[a], *N. Guilbert*[a], *V. Betou*[a], *V.L.M. Esnault*[ab]

Departments of [a]Nephrology, [b]Immunology, [c]Pulmonary Transplantation, Dpts. Nantes University Hospital, France

Extracorporeal photochemotherapy (ECP) has been proposed for the treatment of various auto-immune diseases and allograft rejection in several recent pilot studies. ECP using the Therakos device proved effective in treating and preventing cardiac allograft rejection. To assess efficacy and safety of ECP in pulmonary allograft rejection, we set up a pilot study to treat 5 patients with refractory pulmonary rejection using a new method described by G. Andreu (1). This protocol was approved by our local ethic comittee and is conducted according to good clinical practice.

Five patients with refractory pulmonary rejection will be included in our protocol. Soluble 8-MOP is added ex-vivo to an enriched mononuclear cell suspension obtained by a cell separator (COBE Spectra). This cellular suspension is then irradiated (2J/cm2) using a UV-A irradiator (Vilber Lourmat, Marne La vallée, France) and reinfused to the patient. ECP is performed 2 times a week for 3 weeks, and tapered off according to evolution. The main evaluation criteria is evolution of Forced Expiratory Volume (FEV). Histological examination will be performed on tissue samples obtained from transbronchial biopsy.

Four patients have been included but only two patients completed the first 3 weeks of treatment. We here report the cases of these first two patients treated by ECP in our center. First case report: A 22 year old boy presenting cystic fibrosis received a cardio-pulmonary allogenic transplant in January 1994. One year later he exhibited severe pulmonary rejection with decrease of FEV to a minimum of 69% of theoretical value while Azathioprine had to be stopped because of severe leucopenia. He received 7 ECP treatments in one month. Clinically significant improvement of FEV was observed starting from the second week of treatment (72%) and confirmed at one month (73%). After discontinuing ECP because of lack of vascular access, FEV decreased back to 66%. An arteriovenous fistula has been done to allow further treatments. Second case report: A ll year old girl presenting cystic fibrosis received a cardio-pulmonary allogenic transplant in January 1993. Severe progressive refractory rejection with obliterant bronchiolitis developped with FEV decreasing rapidly from 58 to 48% over 1.5 month. ECP treatment was started without changing immunosuppressive regimen. A stabilization of the FEV has been obtained and she is still currently under treatment. Two other patients have been recently included in this protocol.

ECP treatment using this new device might be a valuable additional treatment for refractory pulmonary rejection. These preliminary results will have to be confirmed at follow-up.

(1) G. Andreu et al. Transfus. Sci. 1994; 15: 443-454

32

Technical Evaluation of a New System for On-Line Hemodiafiltration and Hemofiltration

T. Takagi[a], *T. Uemura*[a], *T Nakatani*[a], *K. Sakurai*[a], *M. Ono*[a], *H. Ogawa*[a], *T. Miyakoda*[b], *K. Uno*[b], *J. Sternby*[b]

[a]Shinsekai daiichi hospital Nagoya
[b]Gambro KK, Japan and Sweden

The performance of a new system of on-line hemodiafiltration and hemofiltration (AK100 ULTRA, Gambro AB, Sweden) has been evaluated concerning a number of key parameters. The study was done as a routine procedure on one machine before starting a clinical study. The parameters studied include the operationability and safety, the residual of disinfectants after rinse, the endotoxin levels, the accuracy and stability of the blood pump flow rate, the dialysate composition and ultrafiltration rate and the dialysate accuracy of the HDF pump flow rate, the heparin pump infusion rate and the temperature control. Flow rates were checked by timed collection, dialysate composition by standard laboratory equipment, and endotoxins by the chromogenic limulus test, Toxicolor system (Seikagaku Kogyo CO LTD, Japan). The blood pump and the HDF pump were both very accurate from 50 ml/min to 500 and 330 ml/min respectively and stable for the 6 hour test. The maximum flow rate error was 3 ml/min at 400 ml/min. Dialysate Sodium was stable for a the 6 hour test, slightly high but always within 2 mEq/l, and bicarbonate was within 1.4 mEq/l. The heparin pump error was less than 0.05 ml/hr from 0.5 to 1.5 ml/hr, and less than 5% at higher flows. The UF control error during 15-30 min was up to 20 ml at set points from 500 to 4000 ml/hr, but the long term stability during 5 hrs at 500 ml/hr was better than 25 ml/hr. Dialysate temperature was about 0.5℃ below set point at normal operating temperature, with a maximum error of 0.87℃ at 39.5℃. The residual level of disinfectant decreased continuously and was below detection limit after less than half of the 40 min rinsing time. Dialysate endotoxin was at the safe level of below 1 pg/ml both before and after the final filter. The main disadvantage with this machine was the maximum dialysate flow rate of 500 ml/min, which is further decreased by the substitution fluid used. This maximum flow has been increased to 700 ml/min in later versions. All the tests performed thus showed satisfactory results so that this machine can be used for clinical trials of on-line HDF.

33

Protein a Immunoadsorption (IA) Reduces Proteinuria in Patients with Nephrotic Syndrome and Membranous Nephropathy

D.P. Besnier[a], *S. Martin*[a], *D. Chabannes*[b], *A. Testa*[a], *P. Simon*[c], *V.L.M. Esnault*[a]

[a]Nephrology and [b]Immunology Departments, Nantes University Hospital
[c]Saint Brieuc Hospital, France

Idiopathic membranous nephropathy (MN) is the main nephrotic syndrome (NS) etiology in adults. Although, association of steroids and cytotoxic drugs may improve long term renal outcome, treatment remains controversial. IA proved to be effective in reducing proteinuria in patients with NS following focal and segmental glomerulosclerosis (FSGS) recurrence on kidney transplant (N.Engl. J. Med. 1994; 330: 7-14). We set up a pilot study to test the effect of IA on proteinuria in 5 patients with NS related to MN. This study was conducted according to the provisions of the Declaration of Helsinki and was approved by the ethic committee of our institution. All participants gave written informed consent.

In order to analyse the specific effect of IA, patients did not receive any concomittent immunosuppressive treatment. Four patients completed the protocol without any major side effect. All four patients exhibited dramatic fall of proteinuria after 5 IA (from 11.6, 13.2, 14.8 and 7.21 g/day respectively to 3.43, 2.94, 2.55 and 1.12 g/day), while serum albumine decreased to a lesser extent (from 27.1, 18.8, 32.1 and 35.6 g/l to 24, 15.6, 23.8 and 23.3 g/l respectively). Proteinuria returned to baseline levels within one week. No adverse side effects were observed.

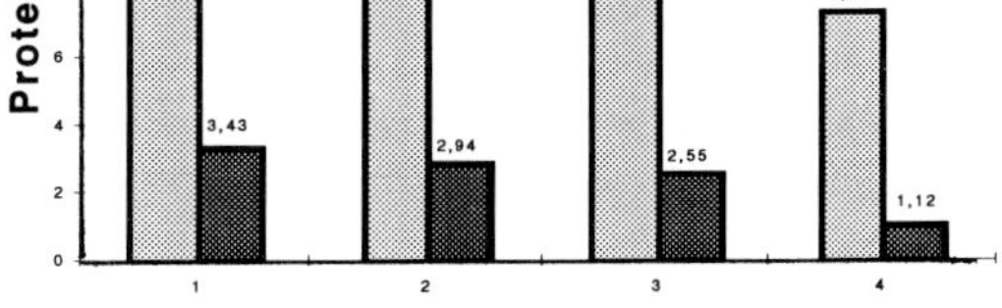

We suggest that IA is effective in producing short term reduction of proteinuria in NS related not only to FSGS but also to MN. A second study, approved by the ethic committee of our institution, is now starting to test the effect of IA in patients presenting NS related to other etiologies. Further studies will test whether immunosupressive drugs are able to prevent the proteinuria rebound observed in these patients.

34

Immunomodulation by Extracorporeal Photochemotherapy (ECP) in Experimental Allergic Encephalomyelitis (EAE)

D. Chabannes[b], D.P. Besnier[a], S. Martin[a], V.L.M. Esnault[ab]

[a]Nephrology and [b]Immunology departments, Nantes University Hospital, France

ECP is a new form of immunomodulatory therapy currently evaluated in several pilot studies in our center. The mechanism of the observed beneficial effect remains unknown. Studies using experimental models suggested that ECP may lead to specific sensitization against pathogenic ECP treated cells. However, no functional basis has been given to its immunomodulatory activity. We studied ECP effect in experimental allergic encephalomyelitis (EAE) in the Lewis rat.

We compared the protective effect of untreated versus ECP-treated encephalitogenic cells on the active induction of EAE in male Lewis rats (8 weeks old) : (a) the active induction of EAE consisted in immunization of the rats with guinea pig spinal cord in complete Freund adjuvant; (b) the encephalitogenic cells were isolated from immunized rats and cultured 3 days with 50 ug/ml of guinea pig myelin basis protein; (c) ECP consisted in UVA irradiation (1.5 J/cm2) in the presence of 8-MOP (100 ng/ml). The recipients (5 rats per group) received 50-70 10^6 of untreated of ECP-treated cells intravenously once a week, and were immunized 7 days later for induction of EAE.

After one month treatment (4 injections) ECP-treated rats were fully protected from the active induction of EAE. The treatment was well tolerated. Rats receiving non-treated cells also showed resistance to active induction of the disease but exhibited EAE symptoms and severe weight loss following the first injection of untreated encephalitogenic cells. Shortening the treatment to one injection revealed that, unexpectedly, ECP treated cells were less efficient in protecting the recipients from the active induction of EAE than the untreated cells. The recipients of untreated cells showed clinical symptoms after the cell transfer but not after immunization. On the other hand, all the recipients of ECP-treated cells, which were perfectly healthy following the transfer, experienced clinical symptoms following immunization. However, these symptoms were less important than in the control group (immunized native rats).

These results suggest that untreated or ECP-treated encephalitogenic effectors are differently handled by the recipients immune system. Untreated cells transferred *passive* EAE, and induced protection against induction of *active* EAE as previously shown. ECP-treated cells were no longer able to transfer *passive* EAE and more than one transfer is necessary to protect the rats from the induction of *active* EAE. Unexpectedly, ECP decreased the potential of encephalitogenic effectors to induce resistance to active EAE since a single transfer of ECP-treated cells appeared inefficient.

35

Clinical Evaluation of Polyflux Dialyzer Membranes

S. Zitta, A. Mauric, J. Roob, H. Holzer

Department of Internal Medicine, Division of Nephrology, University of Graz, Austria

For the treatment of renal failure, high blood compatibility and high removal capacity for middle molecular weight substances are required. This property profile was investigated in a clinical study with Polyamide high-flux dialyzers: polyflux 17 (1.7 m^2), polyflux 21 (2.1 m^2), both ETO-sterilized, and the steam-sterilized polyflux 14"S" (1.4 m^2).

Hemodiafiltration treatments were performed 3 times a week for 3 to 5 hours using a Gambro AK 100 single pass dialysis machine with the HDF 100 weighing system for hemodiafiltraion. Complete recording of the technical parameters was performed with a computerized logging system CCM 100. Whole blood clearances were calculated according to Sternby et al. (Contrib Nephrol 1992; 96: 86-98).

Clearance measurements of urea, phosphate and

Table to Abstract 35

Membrane	urea	phosphate	creatinine	Q_b	UF
polyflux 17	266	262	229	300	67
polyflux 21	290	262	250	352	55
polyflux 14″S"	253	247	230	310	59

creatinine (see table above, values in ml/min) demonstrate the high permeability of the 3 membranes for low-molecular weight substances.

The clearance values did not significantly change during treatment time showing the excellent stability of performance.

Plasma clearance for β_2-microglobulin was found to be 79 (69) ml/min at a mean plasma flow rate of 244 (210) ml/min and a meal UF rate of 55 (56) ml/min for polyflux 21 (polyflux 14″S") membrane.

Leucocyte count (WBC), thrombocyte count and generation of terminal complement complex (TCC) were analyzed as biocompatibility parameters. Low drop in WBC at t = 15 min and no significant change in thrombocyte count over the whole treatment time could be observed. Maximum TCC generation (c_{out}-c_{in} at t = 15 min) was 659 ng/ml, 532 ng/ml and 382 ng/ml for polyflux 17, polyflux 21 and polyflux 14″S", respectively. These data demonstrate that the polyflux dialyzers excert a very low blood/membrane interaction and have a low complement activation potential.

The investigated polyflux membranes are characterized by a three-layer pore-structure, which excerts high and time-constant diffusive and convective permeability for low- and middle- molecular weight substances, but with a sharp cut-off minimizing albumin loss. The hydrophilic/hydrophobic microdomain-structured surface of the membranes leads to low interaction with blood components. Efficient elimination of middle-molecular weight substances and the excellent biocompatibility characteristics of the tested membrances recommend them for acute therapy as well as for long term use in chronic hemodialysis.

36

Randomized Study of Peritoneal Dialysis (PD) Catheter Implantation Using Moncrief (MT) and Conventional Techniques (CT)

Anders Tranæus[a], Anders Danielsson[a], Britta Hylander[b], Linus Blohme[c], RN Christina Eriksson[b], LPN Ewa Malmberg[a]

[a]Department of Nephrology, Huddinge University Hospital

Department of [b]Medicine and [c]Surgery, Karolinska Hospital, Stockholm, Sweden

Background. The Moncrief implantation technique means that the entire PD catheter is placed subcutaneously during ≥ 4 weeks, whereafter the external part is exteriorised operatively. The advantage achieved hereby is thought to be a prevention of early bacterial colonisation/development of biofilm, which might reduce the risk of catheter related infections.

Material. All patients accepted for PD at two major dialysis units, and in which the start of PD was regarded as possible to postpone ≥ 6 weeks were offered participation in the study. All but one accepted. In total 57 patients, were enrolled between September 1992 and March 1995; mean age 60 (31-80) years, 26 women and 15 diabetice (7 MT, 8 CT).

Method. Patients were randomised to either MT or CT. A Moncrief catheter (coiled, swan-neck, extended distal cuff) was implanted laterally with the inner cuff placed in the rectus muscle and the outer cuff subcutaneously. In patients randomised to the CT, the external catheter portion was exteriorized per-operatively. All implantations were performed by two physicians, one at each hospital. Peritonitis (p) and exit-site infections (ESI) were defined according to standard criteria.

Results. All catheters were functioning at start of PD, despite the exclusion of flushing (both groups). The total number of observation months was 495; MT292 and CT203 months. The mean duration from implantation to start of PD was 2 (MT) and 3 (CT) months, respectively. In the MT group 3 episodes of peritonitis occurred (1/97 months) caused by S. aureus, coagulase-negative staphylococci (CONS), and Strep. abdom., respectively, while 6 patients (2 diabetics) in the CT group experienced one episode of p.each (1/34 months), caused by CONS in 3 patients (1 diabetic), enteral organisms, fungi, and streptococci. The incidence of ESI was 1/292 months (MT) and 0/203 months (CT), respectively.

Discussion. This study shows that flushing of the PD catheter post-operatively and during the break-in period is not needed. Furthermore, the low infection rate in both groups might indicate that an extended break-in period (≥ 1 month) is more important that the implantation technique per se.

37

Treatment of Chronic and Acute Graft Versus Host Disease (GvHD) by Extracorporeal Photochemotherapy (ECP) : a Pilot Study

D.P. Besnier[a], D. Chabannes[b], B. Mahé[c], N. Milpied[c], S. Martin[a], N. Guilbert[a], V. Betou[a], V.L.M. Esnault[ab]

Departments of [a]Nephrology, [b]Immunology and [c]Haematology, Nantes University Hospital, France

Extracorporeal photochemotherapy (ECP) has been proposed for the treatment of various auto-immune disease and allograft rejection in several recent pilot studies. GvHD is a major complication following allogenic bone marrow transplantation which may be refractory to immunosuppressive drugs. PUVA therapy has been shown to be effective in treating GvHD skin lesions, and preliminary case reports suggested that ECP using Therakos device may be beneficial. To assess efficacy and safety of ECP in GvHD, we set up a pilot study to treat 5 patients with chronic GvHD (c-GvHD) and 5 with acute GvHD (a-GvHD) using a new method described by G. Andreu (1). This protocol was approved by our local ethical comittee and is conducted according to good clinical practice.

Five c-GvHD and 5 a-GvHD patients will be included in our protocol. Soluble 8-MOP is added ex-vivo to an enriched mononuclear cell suspension obtained by a cell separator (COBE Spectra). This cellular suspension is then irradiated (2J/cm2) using a UV-A irradiator (Vilber Lourmat, Marne La Vallée, France) and reinfused to the patient. ECP is performed 3 times a week for 3 weeks, and tapered off according to evolution. Evaluation includes scoring using Seattle score every days for a-GvHD and specific objective tests for c-GvHD depending on the clinical presentation (quantitative electromyogram, histology...).

We here report the cases of the first two c-GvHD and two a-GvHD patients treated by ECP in our center. The two c-GvHD recovered but not the a-GvHD patients. First c-GvHD case: a 39 year old woman allografted in 1990 following AML was suffering from c-GvHD since 1991. She received steroids, cyclosporine A (CSA) and azathioprine but worserned in August 94 with severe myositis in spite of immunosuppression reinforcement (CSA 150 mg/day, Azathioprine 50 mg/day and Methylprednisolone 48 mg/day) confining her to bed. Muscle biopsy showed evidence of chronic GvHD. After three weeks she was painless, walked normally and exhibited dramatic improvement on electromyogram allowing rapid tapering of immunosuppressive drugs (Methylprednisolone 4 mg/day monotherapy).

Second c-GvHD case: a 13 year old boy developped c-GvHD with mainly skin (hyperalgia) and muscle involvement (bedridden). Rapid improvement after ECP was also observed. a-GvHD cases: the two a-GvHD patients did not modify their liver dysfunctions. However, one patients exhibited cutaneous GvHD lesions which resolved after ECP.

Our protocol of ECP treatment using this new device was effective in c-GvHD, but not in a-GvHD, allowing sparing of immunosuppressive drugs.

(1) G. Andreu et al. Transfus. Sci. 1994; 15: 443-454

38

Treatment of Chronic Progressive Multiple Sclerosis by Extracorporeal Photo-Chemotherary (ECP) : a Pilot Study

D.P. Besnier[a], D. Chabannes[b], J-M. Mussini[a], S. Martin[a], B. Dupas[c], N. Guilbert[a], V. Betou[a], V.L.M. Esnault[ab]

Departments of [a]Nephrology, [b]Immunology, [c]Radiology, Nantes University Hospital, France

Extracorporeal photochemotherapy (ECP) has been proposed for the treatment of various auto-immune diseases and allograft rejection in several recent pilot studies. Multiple sclerosis (MS) is a chronic autoimune disease of the central nervous system presumedly mediated by T cells. Immunosuppressive drugs alter only poorly the course of severe progressive MS with frequent major side effects. To assess the efficacy and safety of ECP in multiply sclerosis, we set up a pilot study to treat 5 patients with chronic progressive form of MS. This protocol was approved by our local ethic committee and is conducted according to good clinical practice.

After giving informed consent, 5 chronic progressive MS patients free of immunosuppression were included in our protocol. Using a method described by G. Andreu (1), soluble 8-MOP is added ex-vivo to an enriched mononuclear cell suspension obtained by a cell separator (COBE Spectra). This cellular suspension is then irradiated (2J/cm2) using a UV-A irradiator (Vilber Lourmat, Marne La vallée, France) and reinfused to the patient. Patients are treated once a week for 6 weeks and then depending on clinical evaluations, for a maximum of 6 months with one year total follow up. Scoring using Kurtzke scale is performed every 6 weeks for the first 6 months, and then every 2 months by a single independant neurologist (J-M.S.). Radiologic follow up with MRI with and without Gadolinium infusion is performed every 6 weeks for the first 6 months and at one year.

Five patients have been included. One patient had to be excluded because of recurrent attack at the very beginning of the treatment. Two patients have already completed the 6 months treatment phase and two others are still under treatment (6 weeks and 4, 5 months). The treatment is well tolerated without any adverse event. The score on Kurtzke scale decreased at the beginning of the treatment and has remained stable since in all patients. No significative changes have been observed so far on MRI analysis. Mononuclear cells collected before and after ECP showed that this treatment abrogate their abality to proliferate in response to mitogenic stimulation.

Our preliminary results may suggest a short term beneficial effect of ECP in the treatment of chronic progressive form of MS, and will have to be confirmed by long term follow-up and larger multicenter studies.

(1) G. Andreu et al. Transfus. Sci. 1994; 15: 443-454

39

The Effect of Ouabain on Peritoneal Transport Characteristics

Park MS[a], Heimburger O[b], Waniewski J[c], Werynski A[c], Lindholm B[b], Lee HB[a]

[a]Hyonam Kidney Laboratory, Seoul, Korea,
[b]Karolinska Institute, Stockholm, Sweden,
[c]Polish Academy of Sciences, Warsaw, Poland

Fluid and solute transport during peritoneal dialysis (PD) is believed to be passive, mainly diffusive and convective transports. Other transport mechanisms than passive transport may, however, also be involved. Intracellular transport of potassium (K) in cultured mesothelial cells is reported to be regulated by a channel that is blocked by Ouabain. High glucose and therefore high insulin in the peritoneal cavity may promote extra to intracellular shift of K during PD.

Aim. To investigate the role of the Ouabain-blocked K channel in peritoneal transport

Methods. A 4-hour single PD was performed in 16 normal Sprague- Dawley rats. Conventional dialysis solution (Dianeal 3.86%®, pH 5.7) containing sufficient K (5.0 ± 0.3 mmol/l) to minimize diffusive transport of K with (PD-O) and without (PD-C) Ouabain (10^{-5}M) was used in 8 rats each. Infusion volume was 30 ml. Intraperitoneal dialysate volume (V_D) was estimated from the dilution of volume marker, ^{131}I human serum albumin (RISA), with corrections for the elimination of RISA from the peritoneal cavity (K_E, ml/min) and sample volume. The diffusive transport coefficient (K_{BD}) and the sieving coefficient (S) were estimated using the modified Babb-Randerson-Farrell model.

Results. D/P of K at the beginning of dialysis was 1.2 ± 0.1. V_D was significantly higher ($p < 0.05$) in PD-O than in PD-C from 120 min of dialysis. K_E (0.058 ± 0.003 vs 0.027 ± 0.018, $p < 0.05$) and fractional amount of glucose absorption were significantly lower in PD-O than in PD-C from 90 min of dialysis. K_{BD} and S values for urea, glucose, sodium and K did not differ between the two solutions.

Conclusions. Ouabain decreased the peritoneal fluid reabsorption (K_E) and peritoneal glucose absorption, and therefore increased V_D. Peritoneal transport of small solutes including K was not influenced by Ouabain during peritoneal dialysis with an acidic dialysis solution in rat.

40

Glucose and Potassium Transport during Experimental Peritoneal Dialysis in Rat

Park MS[a], Heimburger O[b], Waniewski J[c], Werynski A[c], Lindholm B[b], Lee HB[a]

[a]Hyonam Kidney Laboratory, Seoul, Korea, [b]Karolinska Institute, Stockholm, Sweden, [c]Polish Academy of Sciences, Warsaw, Poland

Aim. To investigate characteristics of glucose (G) and potassium (K) transport during experimental peritoneal dialysis (PD).

Methods. A 4-hour single peritoneal dialysis was performed in 14 normal Sprague-Dawley rats. 5% xylitol solution (PD-X, pH 4.7) containing G (118 ± 7 mg/dl) and K (4.9 ± 0.3 mmol/l) to minimize diffusive transport of G and K was used in 7 rats. Conventional dialysis solution (Dianeal 3.86%®, PD-C, pH 5.7) was used in the other 7 rats to provide control values. Infusion volume was 30 ml. Intraperitoneal dialysate volume (V_D) was estimated from the dilution of volume marker, ^{131}I human serum albumin (RISA), with corrections for the elimination of RISA from the peritoneal cavity (K_E, ml/min) and sample volume. The diffusive transport coefficient (K_{BD}) and the sieving coefficient (S) were estimated using the modified Babb-Randerson-Farrell model.

Results. D/P of G and K at the beginning of dialysis were 0.8 ± 0.3 and 1.2 ± 0.1, respectively. V_D was significantly higher in PD-X than in PD-C at 240 min ($p < 0.05$). KE was similar with the two solutions. K_{BD} for G was significantly lower (0.184 ± 0.072 vs 0.325 ± 0.072, $p < 0.05$) and K_{BD} for sodium (Na) was significantly higher (0.246 ± 0.075 vs 0.149 ± 0.079, $p < 0.05$) with PD-X than with PD-C, while K_{BD} for urea and K did not differ between the two solutions. S for G was significantly higher (1.288 ± 0.378 vs 0.037 ± 0.635, $p < 0.05$) and S for Na (0.327 ± 0.149 vs 0.692 ± 0.159, $p < 0.05$) and K (-0.026 ± 0.221 vs 1.14 ± 0.393, $p < 0.05$) were significantly lower with PD-X than with PD-C. S for urea did not differ between the two solutions.

Conclusions. The present findings that S for G and K were anomalous, i.e. out of the range 0-1, with an acidic dialysis solution (PD-X) containing similar concentrations of G and K as in plasma indicate that other transport mechanisms than passive transport is involved in peritoneal transport of G and K.

41

Effect of Prolonged Subcutaneous Implantation of Peritoneal Catheter on Peritonitis Rate during CAPD

Park MS, Lee EY, Cha MK, Kim JH, Song KI, Han DC, Hwang SD, Moon C, Lee HB

Hyonam Kydney Laboratory, Soon Chun Hyang Univiersity, Seoul, Korea

We have previously reported in an uncontrolled study that peritonitis (P) incidence was reduced with the introduction of a new access technique as described by Moncrief in which the external segment of peritoneal catheter was left implanted for 6 weeks before exteriorization and bag exchanges. We, therefore, conducted a prospective randomized controlled study to confirm the earlier observation. Patients who started CAPD between October 1992 and December 1994 and who remained on CAPD for more than 3 mos were included in this analysis. A total of 59 CAPD patients were randomized into 2 groups: 27 patients had catheters inserted by conventional technique (C) and had 6 weeks of break-in period and 32 patients had catheters left implanted subcutaneously for 6 weeks (I). 13 patients (48.1%) from group C and 18 (56.3%) from group I used Y connector (CY and IY) and remaining patients from each group used straight connector (CS and IS). Age, sex and proportion of diabetics were not different between the two groups. The observation period was 264mos for C and 438 mos for I, for a total of 703 mos. The incidence of P was significantly lower in group I compared with group C regardless of connectors (14.8 vs 8.8 mos, $p < 0.05$). The incidence of P was lowest in group IY while this was the highest in group CS (18.1 vs 7.5 mos, $p < 0.05$).

Conclusion. Prolonged subcutaneous implantation of peritoneal catheter significantly reduced the P rate and the use of Y connector further reduced P rate.

42

Incidence of Hypercalcemia in Dialysis Patients: HD vs CAPD

Park MS, Lee EY, Cha MK, Kim JH, Song KI, Han DC, Hwang SD, Lee HB

Hyonam Kidney Laboratary, Soon Chun Hyang University

The use of phosphate (P) binders and high calcium (Ca) dialysate have been standard therapies for dialysis patients. The use of Ca containing phosphate binders, however, has resulted in hypercalcemia in a substantial portion of dialysis population and hence the need for a low Ca dialysis fluid has arisen. In the present study we evaluated the incidence of hypercalcemia among 180 dialysis patients (116 on HD and 64 on CAPD) at Kidney Center, Soon Chun Hyang Univ. Hosp. Dialysate Ca concentrations were 3.0 mEq/L and 3.5 mEq/L for HD and CAPD, respectively. Calcium carbonate was used by 114 HD and 64 CAPD patients and oral calcitriol by 26 HD and 3 CAPD patients. Serum Ca, ionized Ca (iCa), P, albumin (Alb), bicarbonate (HCO_3), alkaline phosphatase (Alk P) were measured monthly and PTH measured once every 6 mos. Total Ca level was corrected by serum albumin level (CCa) and hypercalcemia was defined as CCa over 10.5mg/dl.

None of the patients were hypercalcemic pre-HD while 44 HD patients (37.9%) were hypercalcemic post-dialysis. When pre- and post-HD CCa were averaged, 14 HD patients (12.1%) were hypercalcemic while 5 CAPD patients (7.8%) were found to be hyperclacemic. Average pre- and post-HD CCa (9.7 ± 0.7 mg/dl vs 9.2 ± 0.8 mg/dl, $p < 0.01$) and iCa (1.10 ± 0.11 mmol/L vs 1.05 ± 0.01mmol/L, $p < 0.01$) were significantly higher, and P (4.2 ± 1.0 mg/dl vs 5.0 ± 1.2 mg/dl, $p < 0.01$) significantly lower in HD than in CAPD. Alb (4.0 ± 0.5 mg/dl vs 3.6 ± 0.6 mg/dl, $p < 0.01$) was significantly higher in HD than in CAPD. HCO_3 (18.9 ± 1.8 mmol/L vs 25.2 ± 3.4 mmol/L, $p < 0.01$) was significantly lower in HD than on CAPD. PTH was significantly higher on HD than on CAPD ($p < 0.01$). Alk P did not differ between the two groups. Daily consumption of $CaCO_3$ was higher on HD than on CAPD (2.8 g vs 2.2 g, $p < 0.01$).

In conclusion the incidence of hypercalcemia is high in our HD patients post-dialysis but not pre-dialysis.

43

Dialytic Ultrafiltration (DU) of Ascitic Fluid with Peritoneal Reinfusion of the Concentrate for Refractory Ascites in Patients on Maintanance Hemodialysis (HD)

JM Kong, DS Kang, MK Kim, TD Yoon

Department of Internal Medicine, Maryknoll Hospital, Pusan, Korea

DU of ascitic fluid with peritoneal reinfusion of the concentrate was reported as an effective and safe procedure with no hemodynamic compromise for the treatment of intractable ascites in liver cirrhosis patients (Cadranel JF, Int J Artif Organs 1992). Simple paracentesis may decrease intravascular volume and induce hemodynamic derangement. Colloid infusion along with the paracentesis increases the cost and possibly induces blood borne infection. The protein content in the peritoneally reinfused concentrate seems to enter plasma (Henriksen JH, Scand J Clin Lab Invest 1984), therfore may play a role in stabilizing intravascular volume and also be beneficial nutritionally by avoidance of loss of endogeneous protein.

DU may be an useful procedure for refractory ascites which is resistant to conventional HD in ESRD patients. Fourteen DU were performed on 6 patients on maintanance HD. After heparin free bicarbonate HD, two angiocath plastic cannulas were inserted into the peritoneal cavity on low mid-abdominal line and ascitic fluid was removed by isolated ultrafiltration. The dialyzer used in HD was reused during DU without heparinization. No patients had evidence of liver disease. The fluid volume removed was 2.3 ± 0.7L by HD and 4.1 ± 1.0L of ascites by subsequent DU. Mean arterial pressure, heart rate, plasma renin activity, hematocrit and serum albumin showed no significant changes during HD, during DU and 24 hours thereafter. Plasma ANP fell after HD ($p < 0.05$), but showed no significant change during and up to 24 hours after DU, suggesting no or minimal decrease of intravascular volume by the shifting of fluid from plasma into peritoneal cavity during and up to 24 hours after DU. There was one episode of hemoperitoneum that required blood transfusions, otherwise there were no remarkable complications. In two patients who were noncompliant to fluid restriction DU were repeated at 3.6 ± 1.0 month intervals, but the other 4 patitients required no additional DU during 9.5 ± 1.2 months follow up.

We conclude that DU is an effective and safe procedure with no hemodynamic compromise for the treatment of refractory ascites in HD patients.

44

Plasma Endothelin Concentration during Recombinant Human Erythropoietin (rHuEpo) Administration in Maintenance Hemodialysis Patients

Duk Hee Kang, Kyu Bok Choi, Kyun Il Yoon

Department of Internal Medicine, College of Medicine, Ewha Women's University Hospital, Seoul, Korea

The pathogenesis of hypertension occurring during correction of anemia with rHuEpo in end stage renal disease patients still remains unclear. Endothelial cells have receptors for rHuEpo and release of endothelin (ET), one of th most potent vasoconstrictor, with endothelial damage. Although several studies revealed the possible link of rHuEpo treatment and ET release, there were discordant data about rHuEpo-induced hypertension and plasma ET concentration. The present study was undertaken to evaluate the correlation between changes in plasma ET concentration and an increase of blood pressure during rHuEpo administration in 14 hemodialysis patients (M:F 8:6) with the measurement of hemodynamic parameters. rHuEpo was started at a dose of 2000 unit, given subcutaneously two or three times a week, at the end of each dialysis session. Various parameters including hematocrit (Hct), erythropoietin and endothelin concentration were measured before treatment and two weeks interval during the first eight weeks of rHuEpo. We also evaluated stroke volume (SV), cardiac index (CI) and total peripheral vascular resistance (TPVR) by doppler echocardiography before and eight weeks after rHuEpo.

Mean Hct and erythropoietin level before rHuEpo was 20.4±6.7% and 5.5±2.1mU/ml respectively, and started to increase significantly 2 weeks after rHuEpo. Plasma ET concentration before rHuEpo was 2.9±1.2 pg/ml, and there was no significant correlation between ET level and systolic or diastolic blood pressure. No significant changes in plasma ET were found during rHuEpo.

After eight weeks of rHuEpo, SV (58.4±7.3 vs. 49.7 ±6.5 ml/m^2, $p < 0.01$) and CI (4.22±0.66 vs. 3.17± 0.71 L/min/m^2, $p < 0.05$) decreased significantly with an increase of TPVR (1223±51 vs. 1719±34 dyn.sec/cm^5, $p < 0.01$). An elevation in blood pressure was found in four patients (28.6%). In these rHuEpo-induced hypertension group, absolute value of ⊿SV before and eight weeks after rHuEpo was significantly lower compared to the group without rHuEpo-induced hypertension (9.8±4.1 vs 1.7±5.4, $p < 0.01$) in spite of no significant differences of ⊿Hct, ⊿erythropoietin, ⊿ET and ⊿TPVR according to the presence of rHuEpo-induced hypertension. In conclusion, rHuEpo-induced hypertension was not related with the rate of Hct increase, erythropoietin and endothelin concentration during rHuEpo administration. The most important factor which distinguished those patients whose blood pressure rised from the remainder was a failure of stoke volume to fall. Therefore volume status of patients should be carefully monitored with correction of anemia with rHuEpo in hemodialysis patients.

Table to Abstract 44

	0 week	2 week	4 week	8 week
Hct (%)	20.4±6.7	24.7±7.2*	28.9±6.7*	30.1±5.1*
Erythropoietin (mU/ml)	5.5±2.1	6.4±3.2*	6.9±1.4**	8.2±3.4**
Endothelin (pg/ml)	2.9±1.2	3.0±2.1	2.9±1.5	3.4±6.9

* ; $p < 0.05$ vs. 0 week value, ** ; $p < 0.05$ vs. 2 week value

45

Plasma Concentrations and Productions of IL-1, TNF α and IL-6 by Peripheral Blood Mononuclear Cells (PBMC) in Chronic Hemodialyzed Patients

JH Ahn[b], JK Park[a], YH Kim[a], TW Lee[a], CG Ihm[a] & MJ Kim[a]

[a]Department of Internal Medicine, Kyung Hee Univ. Hospital

[b]Kyung Hee Cha Hospital, Seoul, Korea

To evaluate the effect of hemodialysis membrane on cytokine production, we measured the pre- and post-dialysis plasma concentrations of IL-1, TNFα, IL-6 and their productions by 24-hours cultured PBMC (1) in cases of chronic dialysis with polymethyl-methacrylate (group PMMA1) (2) in patients switched into cuprophan for 6 times (group Cuprophan) and (3) after further 6times of dialysis with PMMA again (group PMMA2). Plasma IL-1 concentration in pre-PMMA1 (45.32 ± 2.63 fmol/ml) was significantly high compared to that of normal control subjects (33.81 ± 2.38 fmol/ml) ($p < 0.05$). Plasma IL-1 concentration in pre-PMMA2 (40.21 ± 3.16 fmol/ml) was significantly low compared to those of pre-PMMA1 (45.32 ± 2.63 fmol/ml: $p < 0.01$) and pre-Cuprophan (43.74 ± 3.57 fmol/ml: $p < 0.05$). IL-1 productions by PBMC in pre-Cuprophan (29.77 ± 6.18 fmol/ml) and pre-PMMA2 (25.36 ± 3.53 fmol/ml) were low compared to that in pre-PMMA1 (46.88 ± 7.33 fmol/ml) (both $p < 0.05$). IL-6 production by PBMC in pre-PMMA2 (264.8 ± 60.8 fmol/ml) was low compared to pre-PMMA1 (604.0 ± 78.5 fmol/ml) ($p < 0.05$). There were significant correlations between IL-1 and TNFα ($r = 0.59$, $p < 0.001$), IL-1 and IL-6 ($r = 0.69$, $p < 0.001$), TNFα and IL-6 ($r = 0.59$, $p < 0.001$) in the productions by PBMC. In conclusion, IL-1, TNFα and IL-6 are produced interrelatedly by PBMC in chronic hemodialyzed patients. The productions of these cytokines by PBMC may by induced by long-term, not short-term, stimulations with same dialysis membrane without regard to membrane types.

46

Study of Membrane Biocompatibility in Chronic Hemodialysis Patients

YH Lee. MK Chang, NH Kim, SK Cho, YS Kim JR Koo, DR Cha, YJ Kwon, WY Cho, HK Kim

Department of Internal Medicine, Korea University, Seoul, Korea

Purpose. It is well known that chronic renal failure patients undergoing hemodialysis have several indices of immune deficiency. And the effect of hemodialysis on immune status of the patients may be associated with the biocompatibility of the dialysis membrane. The magnitude of the changes in a blood constituents on exposure to the dialysis membrane has been used as an index of biocompatibility.

Methods. To evaluate the influence of different dialysis membrane, Cuprophane membrane and polymethylmethacrylate (PMMA) membrane, on the immune status of the chronic renal failure patients on hemodialysis, prospective crossover design study was performed on 15 patients receiving chronic hemodialysis with PMMA membrane for 17 months. All the patient included in the study were chronic renal failure patients and had no systemic disease affecting immune status of the patients. Study was performed in 3 phase. In phase I patients were dialysed with Cuprophan membrane for 5 weeks, in phase II the patients were switched to 5 weeks of PMMA membrane dialysis and then they were returned to 5 weeks of Cuprophane membrane dialysis in phase III. Blood samples for various indices of immune status of the patients were obtained at the beginning and end of each phase. Control blood samples were obtained from 10 healthy adults. The results are as follows.

Results. (1) Serum β_2-microglobulin levels in patient group were significantly elevated than in the normal control group (28.32 ± 11.18 vs 1.17 ± 0.18 μg/dl, $p < 0.05$). In phase I and phase III, there are significant ($p < 0.05$) elevation of serum β_2-microglobulin, namely from 28.32 ± 11.28 to 31.89 ± 8.38 and from 35.00 ± 11.29 to 38.27 ± 12.42 μg/dl, respectively. But in phase II, dialysis with PMMA membrane, there was no significant change in serum β_2-microglobulin level. (2) Serum soluble interleukin-2 receptor (sIL-2R) levels were markedly elevated in patient group (1564 ± 712 vs 495 ± 105 U/ml, $p < 0.05$). There were significant elevation of sIL-2R level in phase I and phase III, from 1564 ± 713 to 1928 ± 542 in phase I and from 1744 ± 508 to 1958 ± 634 U/ml in phase III. But in phase II, serum sIL-2R level did not change significantly. (3) There were no significant differences of interleukin-2 receptor (IL-2R) expression on peripheral lymphocyte between patient group and normal control. Also there were no significant changes of IL-2R expression according to dialysis membrane. (4) Other immunologic parameters, serum C_3 level, T_4/T_8 cell ratio and NK/T cell ratio are decreased significantly in patient group. But there are no significant changes in serum level according to each phase.

Conclusions. Above results suggest that PMMA membrane may be more biocompatible than Cuprophan membrane, because PMMA membrane results in less elevation in β_2-microglobulin and sIL-2R. But further study is required.

47

Effects of Dialysis Membranes on Beta 2-Microglobulin (β_2M)

YJ Kwon, NH Kim, SK Cho, KS Wee, YS Kim, JR Ku, DR Cha, WY Cho, HJ Pyo, HK Kim

Department of Internal Medicine, Korea University, Seoul, Korea

Retention of β_2M in patients undergoing hemodialysis is associated with a β_2M-derived amyloidosis. Main pathogenesis of retention of β_2M in ESRD patients is loss of residual renal function. The role that the biocompatibility of dialysis membrane plays in the generation of β_2M has been controversial. To eveluate the effects of different dialysis membranes on serum β_2M change and β_2M production by peripheral blood mononuclear cells (PBMC), we measured serum β_2M & the vitro production of β_2M by PBMC harvested from 8 chronic hemodialysis patients (M:F = 5:3, mean age: 39.4 ± 10.2 years) after dialysis with different membranes : Cuprophane & polymethylmethacrylate (PMMA) dialyzer.

Methods. (1) The design of the study was 2 phase. During the first phase of the study all pateints were dialyzed each time with cuprophane membrane. The patients were switched to 2 months of PMMA membranes without other changes in dialysis parameters. Blood samples were drawn pre-& post- dialysis monthly and measured by RIA. (2) PBMC were collected by Ficoll-Histopaque method and incubated in non-saturated- & dialysis membrane- saturated- serum free media (RPMI 1640) for 5 hrs. Supernatants were measured by RIA.

Results. (1) The concentration of serum β_2M at pre-HD was decreased after change of dialysis membrane from cuprophane to PMMA. (26.93 ± 1.28 vs 24.36 ± 1.21, 23.53 ± 1.14, $p < 0.05$). (2) The release of β_2M by PBMC was increased in each dialysis membrane-saturated- media. (nonsaturaed vs. cuprophane vs. PMMA 9.3% vs. 15.6% vs. 20.9%, $p > 0.05$).

Conclusion. The serum β_2M concentrations were decreased after change of dialysis membrane from cuprophane to PMMA. The results may be caused not by the effects of dialysis membrane on β_2M release by PBMC, but by the dialyzable effect of membrane on β_2M.

48

Effect of Endotoxin Adsorption on Plasma Amino Acids in Severe Sepsis

Shigeru Kanesaka, Yoshiki Takahashi, Kazuhide Iizuka, Tadao Akizawa

Fujigaoka Hospital, Showa University, Yokohama

Purpose. Plasma pattern of amino acids is known as a marker for tissue metabolism.

We had reported the improvement of mean arterial pressure and systemic vascular resistance index by endotoxin adsorption with polymyxin B immobilized fiber (Toraymyxin: Toray, Tokyo).

This study focused to the influence of Toraymyxin on plasma amino acids in septic patients.

Methods. Severe sepsis on the definitions of systemic inflammatory response syndrome was diagnosed in 19 patients including 11 cases with renal and/or hepatic dysfunction.

Table to Abstract 48

nmol/ml	before	after	p
Asparagine	36 ± 13	42 ± 13	< 0.05
Glutamine	328 ± 96	372 ± 106	< 0.01
Proline	107 ± 40	136 ± 56	< 0.01
Alanine	245 ± 68	301 ± 85	< 0.01
Valine	171 ± 30	197 ± 42	< 0.01
Cysteine	46 ± 26	54 ± 28	< 0.01
Isoleucine	44 ± 13	52 ± 14	< 0.01
Leucine	101 ± 15	122 ± 24	< 0.01
Tyrosine	60 ± 15	70 ± 18	< 0.01
Phenylalanine	128 ± 46	142 ± 42	< 0.01
Arginine	54 ± 13	64 ± 11	< 0.05
Fisher's ratio	1.75 ± 0.53	1.84 ± 0.55	

The adsorption was performed 12 times in 9 survivors and 13 times in 10 nonsurvivors.

Plasma levels of amino acids were examined before and after the adsorption.

Results. mean ± SD in 9 survivors.

These changes were almost same in 10 nonsurvivors but not significant except phenylalanine ($p < 0.05$).

Conclusions. The plasma pattern of amino acids other than cysteine and phenylalanine could be normalized. It indicated that Toraymyxin would be useful for the improvement of tissue metabolism in septic patients.

49

Elution of Polymorphonuclear Cells and Lymphocytes from Dialyzers: Lymphocytes as a Novel Index of Bioincompatibility

MPC Grooteman[a], MJ Nubé[a], AJ van Houte[a], J van Limbeek[b]

[a]Medical Center Alkmaar, Departments of Hemodialysis and Immunology

[b]Municipal Health Centre Amsterdam

During hemodialysis (HD), enhanced adhesion and degranulation of polymorphonuclear cells (PMN) has been observed in peripheral blood (PB). In addition, activation of lymphocytes (Ly) and Ly-subset changes also occur. Although manifestations of bio-incompatibility (BI) are usually studied in PB, BI originates in the dialyzer itself. Hence, we developed a dialyzer elution technuque, as has been described before, in order to analyze cells adherent to the membrane.

In the present study, Ly and PMN were analyzed in dialyzer eluates (DE) and PB after 3 hours of routine HD. Eight patients were randomized to cellulose triacetate (CTA), polysulfon (PS) and cuprammonium (CU) membranes in a cross-over design. Leukocyte count and light microscopic differentiation were performed in DE and PB. Furthermore, the expression of the degranulation markers CD63 and CD66b (CD67), and the adhesion marker CD62L on PMN, as well as Ly-subsets (T: CD3, B: CD19, and NK-cells: CD16/56) were assessed by flow cytometry.

Eluates contained 53 x 10^6 cells on average. Microscopic differentiation showed mainly PMN (87%), differing significantly from PB (69%, $p < 0.001$), while relatively few Ly were found (DE 7% vs PB 24%, $p < 0.001$). The expression of degranulation markers was considerably higher on PMN in DE than in PB: mean fluorescence intensity (MFI) of CD66b: DE 2302 and PB 306, $p = 0.003$. In contrast, CD62L was down-regulated in DE: MFI 377 and PB 3688, $p = 0.001$. Both degranulative and adhesive activity on PMN were similar for all membranes. Ly-subpopulations in DE from CTA and CU were comparable to PB. However, PS DE showed a markedly different pattern: more B (22% vs 6%, $p = 0.05$) and NK-cells (30% vs 16%, $p = 0.03$), but fewer T-cells (37% vs 78%, $p < 0.001$).

From these data, it appears that: (1) the majority of eluted cells were PMN. (2) eluted PMN showed substantial enhanced degranulative activity, significantly different from PB, but similar for all three membranes. (3) Ly adherence appears to be non-selective (= similar to PB) in case of cellulosic membranes, but selective in case of PS. (4) in dialyzer eluates, Ly might represent a novel and better parameter for the evaluation of BI as compared with PMN.

50

Clinical Analysis of Patients with Multiple Organ Failure Treated with Plasmapheresis

M. Kihara, S. Yuasa, T. Sumikura, N. Takahashi, T. Shouji, K. Uchida, H. Fujioka and H. Matsuo

The 2nd Department of Internal Medicine, Kagawa Medical School, Kagawa, Japan

It has been generally assumed the multiple organ failure (MOF) is characterized by a poor prognosis. In this study, we examined the clinical characteristics of patients with MOF and the efficacy of plasmapheresis (PP) in those patients. Forty patients with MOF who were treated with PP at the Kagawa Medical School Hospital between April 1989 and December 1994 were studied. They included 25 men and 15 women. Ages ranged from 22 to 84 years, with a mean of 56.5. MOF was diagnosed when a patient had two or more failed organs simultaneously according to the following criteria: (1) respiratory failure: respiration supported by a respirator: (2) hepatic failure: serum total bilirubin level > 5 mg/dl or hepaplastin test < 40%: (3) cardiac failure: inotoropic support required to maintain blood pressure: (4) renal failure: serum creatinine > 3 mg/dl and/or urine output of < 400 ml/day: (5) central nervous system disorder: responding only to deep pain: (6) gastrointestinal bleeding: bleeding requiring blood transfusion: and (7) DIC: DIC score > 7. The most frequent fundamental disease were liver disease, malignant neoplasm and heart disease. Twenty two patients received surgery and subsequently developed MOF. Plasma exchange (PE) was carried out in 23 patients and plasma absorption (PA) in 9 patients. The remaining 8 patients received PE and PA combined therapy. In 14 patients with renal failure, hemodialysis (HD) and/or hemofiltration (HF) were also required. Among the 40 patients, 35 died, so the mortality in this population was 87.5%. Except one patient, all who had liver disease and malignant neoplasm died. Of the 7 failed organs evaluated, hepatic failure, renal failure and DIC were frequently observed. There were 15 cases combining hepatic failure and renal failure, and 13 cases combining hepatic failure, renal failure and DIC in the interrelationships of failed organs. The mortalities of the patients with hepatic failure, renal failure and DIC were 89%, 85% and 53%, respectively. From these results, it has been considered that measures to treat liver disease and postoperative management are of importance to prevent MOF. Furthermore, an organic correlation between renal failure, hepatic failure and DIC was speculated. Further treatment devices are necessary in patients with MOF.

51

Simplified Calculation for G and nPCR by 2 Points Bun Measurement AT Pre-And Post-Hemodialysis

Ichiro Nakagawa[a], Hisao Urano[a], Yutaka Koda[b], Masashi Suzuki[b], Yoshihei Hirasawa[b]

[a]Kidney Center of shinrakuen Hospital, Clinical engineering section, [b]Internal Medicine. Niigata, Japan

Purpose. Since maintenance hemodialysis (HD) system was instituted in 1968 in our hospital, BUN was measured at pre- and post- first HD of a week regularly. Our aim was to make it possible to calculate G and nPCR from the past data, lacking BUN at pre-midweek HD, by a widely-used spreadsheet software on a personal computer.

Methods. Subjects were 180 anuric stable patients on maintenance HD in our hospital in whom same dialysis was done thrice weekly. V at dry weight was determined by Hume's formula (1971). Pre- and post-BUN values were simulated with using BUN reduction rate (RR) of first HD, dialysis time, body weight, gender and amount of removed fluid. The calculations were $C3 = (G \cdot t + C2 \cdot V) / (V + dBW)$, $C4 = C3 \cdot (1 - RR)$, where C3 and C4 were pre-and post-BUN of 2nd HD. RR was corrected by changed V when calculating 2nd and 3rd HD BUN. Appropriate G was determined by iteration till $|C1 - C7| < 0.01$ mg/dl on spreadsheet (C1: pre-BUN of 1st HD, C7: pre-BUN of 1st HD next week). Calculated parameters were compared with measured parameters (3 points method).

Results. G and nPCR by our 2 points method and those by 3 points method did not differ significantly (paired-t test). nPCR (g/kg/day) was 1.26 ± 0.26 vs 1.26 ± 0.27 and G (mg/min) 5.57 ± 1.68 vs 5.58 ± 1.63 (2 vs 3 points method).

Conclusions. Although some restrictions exist, our simplified method is useful in calculating nPCR from the past data of 2 points, and can be done easily by a spreadsheet on a personal computer.

52

Iliopsoas Bursitis is a Rare Complication Associated with Beta-2 Microglobulin (β_2M) Amyloid in Longterm Hemodialysis Patients

Yutaka Koda[a], Shigeru Miyazaki[a], Yasuko Yuasa[a], Masashi Suzuki[a], Yoshihei Hirasawa[a], Takashi Morita[b], Takeshi Kamura[c]

Kidney Center of Shinrakuen Hospital, [a]Internal Medicine and [b]Pathology

[c]Radiology of Niigata University, Niigata, Japan

Purpose. Iliopsoas bursitis is a rare and secondary manifestation usually of rheumatoid or osteoarthritis of the hip. We observed this bursitis in 3 cases of long-term hemodialysis (HD) patients and found the association with β_2-M amyloid.

Cases. Their ages were 43 to 78 years old, 2 males and 1 female and 9 to 21 years on HD. The presenting symptoms were inguinal mass, pain in all cases and fever in one. They all had carpal tunnel syndrome due to β_2M amyloid. Two patients showed clear bone cyst on X-ray in femoral neck. CT scan showed low dense mass in iliopaoas muscle compressing femoral vein

medially. Magnetic Resonance Imaging (MRI) showed large cyst over hip joint extending under inguinal ligament and anterior upper thigh. Yellow mucinous fluid was aspirated by puncture and materials stained with Congo-red, with apple-green birefringence under polarized light were found in it.

Conclusions. Iliopsoas bursitis is a rare and a new type of complication of β_2M amyloid. If should be one of the important differential diagnoses of a painful swelling in the inguinal region in long-term HD patients. CT scan and MRI are very helpful for the diagnosis.

53

Pseudomonas Peritonotis in Patients on CAPD

S.K. Jo, Y.J. Kwon, N.H. Kim, M.K. Chang, K.S. Wee, J.R. Koo, D.R. Cha, W.Y. Cho, H.J. Pyo, H.K. Kim

Department of Internal Medicine, Korea University Seoul, Korea

Purpose. Pseudomonas infection is still unnoticed as the important cause of peritonitis in patients in patients on CAPD. While it accounts for less than 20% of cases, it contributes significantly to the morbidity and mortality in our centers. We report our center's experience of 22 episodes of pseudomonas peritonitis comparing with methicillin-resistant Stapylococcus aureus (MRSA) about their risk factors and prognosis, and also investigated the factors that determine the prognosis of pseudomonas peritonitis.

Method. (1) We analysed 22 episodes of pseudomonas peritonitis occuring in 20 patients, out of 115 patients managed on CAPD from December 1989 to March 1995 in Korea- University- Hospital comparing with MRSA group about their risk factors and overall prognosis. (2) We investigated the factors that influence the prognosis of pseudomonas peritonitis such as organisms, the duration of antibiotics and degree of antibiotics resistance.

Result 1. (1) There were 146 cases of peritonitis which cultures were positive. Of 146 episodes of peritonitis, pseudomonas accounts for 22%, MRSA 19%, methicillin-sensitive Staphylococci 30% and fungal infection 10%. (2) The occurence of complication, such as ascites, subsequent fungal infection is found only in pseudomonas group. (3) The sex, age, underlying disease, the glucose concentration in dialysate solution, number of preceding peritonitis and exitsite infection did not differ significantly between the two groups. (4) In pseudomonas peritonitis, the frequency of catheter removal is significantly higher than in MRSA group.

Result 2. (1) Pseudomonas aeruginosa was dominant in poor prognosis group (80%). (2) The degree of antibiotics resistance, the duration of antibiotics therapy did not influence the prognosis significantly.

Conclusion. Pseudomonas peritonitis usually has a more severe and prolonged course than other bacterial peritonitis and it often cannot be controlled without catheter removal despite antibiotics treatment. So, in the case of pseudomonas peritonitis, early catheter removal can by considered carefully because it can improve the longterm prognosis of the patients on CAPD.

54

Endotoxin Contamination in Reverse Osmosis-Treated Water and Dialysate - A Multi Center Study

Shaw-Yih Liou, Mei-Pu Lin, Chi-Lin Chang, Tzay-Jinn Chen

Society of Blood Purification R.O.C

Throughout the process of each hemodialysis session, each patient's blood will be in contact with at least 100 liters of dialysate. Should dialysate be contaminated with endotoxin, endotoxin could be transferred to patient's blood stream via back filtration and induced cytokine formation, which leads to various osmosis-treated water and diluted dialysate from 23 dialysis centers in Taipei and Tainan metropolitan. The endotoxin levels were examined with kinetic QCL method. The result showed that the average endotoxin concentrations of 0.21 ± 0.4 EU/ml in RO-treated water and 0.77 ± 0.84 EU/ml in diluted dialysate ($p = 0.0063$). R.O. treated water and diluted dialysate from few dialysis centers showed significant endotoxin contamination. In general, the level of endotoxin is higher in diluted dialysate than in R.O. treated water. These findings prompt us to conclude that bicarbonate dialysate can easily be contaminated by endotoxin. Therefore susceptibility of bicarbonate dialysate to microbial and/or endotoxin contamination deserve our serious attention.

55

Effect of Epimedium Sagittatum on Quality of Life and Cellular Immunity in Patients on Maintained Hemodialysis

Xiang-Mei Chen, Hong-Jun Liao.
Departmemt of Nephrol, General Hospital of PLA, Beijing, PRC

In our previous study, Chinese medicine Epimedium Sagittatum (EP) was demonstrated to be of immunoenhance effect on the animal model of chronic renal insufficiency. In present study, we studied the therapeutic effect and the immune regulation capacity of EP on maintained hemodialysis patients. 34 cases of regular hemodialysis patients were divided into 2 groups. Group 1 was treated with EP in form of decoction for 4 months, and 25 healthy donors were taken as normal control. The clinical manifestations and interleukin-2 (IL-2), soluble interleukin-2 receptor (sIL-2R) and interleukin-6 (IL-6) were investigated monthly. It was found that EP had sexual potentitation effect and improved the quality of life in patients of chronic renal failure on regular hemodialysis. The production of IL-2 by peripheral lymphocytes increased siginficantly ($p < 0.01$) in Group 1. The level of sIL-2R elevated significantly, while the level of IL-6 decreased markedly in Group 2 ($p < 0.01$). But the level of sIL-2R and IL-6 restored to normal level in Group 1. The results suggested that Chinese medicine EP has therapeutic effect on sexual disorders and immune regulation capacity in patients of chronic renal failure undergoing hemodialysis.

56

Evaluation of The Dialytic Efficiency by KT/V Urea Modelling in High-Flux Hemodialysis (HFD)

Xiang-Mei Chen, Ning Zhu
Department of Nephrology, General Hospital of PLA, Beijing, PRC

To evaluate the efficiency of HFD based on kinetic modelling of urea, 11 patients (8 males and 3 females) with a dialysis duration < 6 months of conventional hemodialysis (HD) were switched to HFD for 2 months. 5 cases treated twice a week and 6 patients was three times a week. Fresenius A-2008D machine and Fresenius F60 dialysers were used. HFD was 3 hrs and with dialytic blood flow individualized in a range of 300-380 ml/min.

Results. the KT/V value was higher in HFD than that in HD (1.3 ± 0.3 vs 1.1 ± 0.3, $p < 0.05$). KT/V was showed to be of no related with the time of each HD, but related to the blood flow. There was no difference of KT/V in comparision between 2/week and 3/week HD patients, while KT/V per week was higher in the patients with 3/week HD and HDF than those of 2/week HD and HFD patients ($p < 0.01$). The KT/V per week was higher in those with survival renal function (SRF) than those without SRF ($p < 0.05$). There was a significant correlationship between protein catabolic rate and KT/V ($p < 0.01$).

Conclusion. The results suggested that patients undergoing HFD and regular HD should receive KT/V monitoring in order to improve the survival quality.

57

A Survey of the Nutritional Status of Patients Undergoing Chronic Hemodialysis

Mei-hua Zhou, Xiang-mei Chen
Department of Nephrol, General Hospital of PLA, Beijing, PRC

Almost all those uremic patients undergoing chronic hemodialysis (HD) suffer from a long-term progressive dystrophy. The morbidity of patients on maintained HD and the episodes of dialysis complications are closely related to the nutritional status of the HD patients. In order to decrease the frequency of complications and to prolong the survival time of the patients, we studied the nutritional status in 35 uremic patients (24 males and 11 females, age range 18~71 yo, HD duration 1~11 months, mean duration 6.1 ± 3.2 months) on maintained HD. PMMA dialysers (Toray, Japan) and bicarbonate dialysate were applied for 2~3 dialysis (4~5 hr/dialysis) each week. Kt/V value and TACurea were used to ascertain sufficient dialysis. The results indicate that those with insufficient protein intake account for 57.1% (20/35, $p < 0.01$), and 77.1% (27/35) patients showed an insufficient intake of calorie ($p < 0.01$). All the patients showed an extremely insufficient intake of vitamins and minerals (including trace elements). 28.6% (10/35) patients showed a moderate dystrophy, and 40.0% (14/35) patients showed a mild dystrophy. All the patients showed a marked decrease of serum level of amino acids, transferrin, prealbumin and albumin. Conclusionally, all the 35 patients serveyed in this study suffered from a long-term dystrophy. And futhermore, the dialysis staff should give the patients dietary guidance, thus to improve the quality of life, to prolong the survival time of the HD patients.

58

Expression of Interleukin 8 (IL-8), IL-1 Beta and IL-6 mRNA in Hemodialysis (HD) Patients

Hong-Jun Liao, Xiang-Mei Chen, Shu-Wen Liu

Department of Nephrol, General Hospital of PLA, Beijing, PRC

The expression of mRNA from peripheral blood mononuclear cells pre-and 1hr post-HD, derived from 5 HD patients dialyzed with new dialyzers of Cuprophan membrane, were measured by using synthesized oligonucleotide primers of human IL-8, IL-1 beta and IL-6 for cytokine mapping. For semiquantitative analysis of mRNA, aliquots (10ul) were taken after every 4 cycles from 16 to 36th, analyzed on 1.5% agarose gels and PCR products were stained with ethidium bromide. The results showed that the cycle number of PCR product signal of IL-8 (5/5), IL-1 beta (3/5) and IL-6 (3/5) were occurred 4 to 8 cycles earlier and stronger in 1hr HD than those pre-HD. It was suggested that there were increased gene expression of these cytokines after 1hr HD and IL-8 might be as a marker for detection of biocompatibility of dialyzer membrane.

59

Biocompatibility of dialyzer Membranes: Comparision of Four Kinds of Hemodialysis Membranes

Xiang-Mei Chen, Ning Zhu

Department of Nephrol, General Hospital of PLA, Beijing, PRC

To evaluate the biocompatibility of dialyzer membrane, four kinds of membranes including cuprophan (Cu), cellulose acetate (CA), Hemophan (HP) and polymethylmetharcylate (PMMA) were used sequentially in the same patient. Eleven patients (8 males and 3 females, mean age 46 ± 12 yo) were investigated and the white blood cell (WBC) count, plasma C3, interleukin 1 (IL-1), IL-6 and tumor necrosis factor alpha (TNFα) were selected as the biocompatibility parameters. The results showed: A marked leukopenia was observed at 30, 60 min. of hemodialysis using cuprophan dialyzers, and a markedly increased plasma C3 at 60 min. Neither WBC nor C3 showed significant changes when CA, HP and PMMA dialyzers were used. There was a significant elevation of IL-1 patients of one hour HD using Cu, CA and HP dialyzers. Serum IL-1 didn't increase in those using PMMA dialyzers. Serum TNFα elevation was observed in patients using all four kinds of dialyzers, and a significant increase was found in those using Cu and CA dialyzers. Serum IL-6 was found to be not modified by HD performed with any kind of the membranes. In conclusion, PMMA dialyzer shows the best biocompatibility, the next is HP and CA dialyzers, and the cuprophan dialyzer is not well-biocompatable.

60

β_2-Microglobulin (β_2-M) Removal with Different Blood Purification Extracorporeal Methods

R. Marangoni, R. Savino, F. Masi, A. Manfredi, R. Cimino, R. Colombo, L. Maltagliati, G. Romei Longhena

Nephrology and Dialysis Unit, Bollate Hospital-Mi, Italy

Even if the role of β_2-M in amyloidosis pathogenesis in chronic uremic patients undergoing regular dialysis is not clear yet, its degree removal is however an important parameter of the blood purification method efficiency in eliminating large molecules. Therefore we wanted to study β_2-M removal with different blood purification methods and more precisely with: (a) Acetate Free Biofiltration (AFB), exploiting convection and diffusion simultaneously. (b) High Efficiency Paired Filtration Dialysis (HEPFD), i.e. hemofiltration + hemodialysis in series, therefore exploiting convection and diffusion separately. (c) Hemofiltration (HF) with two different membranes: hydrophilic poliamide (PA)

Table to Abstract 61

	CHD	CAPD	P
number	42	45	N.S.
$25OHD_3$ (nmol/L)	39.9 ± 19.7	13.4 ± 14.6	< 0.0001
1.25 $(OH)_2D_3$ (pmol/L)	22.3 ± 14.4	17.2 ± 16.7	< 0.03

and polisulfone (PS) (d) HF (with PA and PS) + hemoperfusion (with collodion-coated activated charcoal, CAC) in series (HF+HP).

With each of these methods (in HF and HF+HP with each of the two membranes employed) we treated 6 chronic anuric uremic patients for 6 months. All these patients were treated previously with bicarbonate dialysis (4 hours, 3 times weekly, cuprophan) for 6 months. In the treated patients we determined: (a) β_2-M clearance of each method (and membrane) employed. (b) the amount of β_2-M removed in only one treatment of each method (and membrane) except HF+HP, because of the impossibility of determining the amount of β_2-M adsorbed by CAD. (c) serum predialytic values of β_2-M before the beginning of the new treatment and after 6 months.

The obtained results show: (a) β_2-M clearance (mean values determined after 60 min from the treatment starting) is very high in HF+HP (156 ml/min with PA and 147 ml/min with PS), is high in HF (90 ml/min with PA and 74 ml/min with PS), lower in HEPFD (60 ml/min) and very low in AFB (43 ml/min). (b) β_2-M removed in one session shows the same trend: 300 mg in HF with PA, 286 mg in HF with PS, 180 mg in HEPFD, 102 mg in AFB. (c) β_2-M serum level modifications after 6 months are in accordance with the above mentioned results: the decrease of β_2-M serum concentrations is highly significant ($p < 0.001$) in patients treated with HF+HP, slightly significant ($p < 0.05$) in patients treated with HF: no significant in patients treated with HEPFD and AFB. Therefore, among the usual extracorporeal blood purification methods, HF shows to be the most efficient method in β_2-M removal, but only HP addition (HF+HP) can give so high removal as to warrant a β_2-M negative balance.

61

The Elimination of Vitamin D with CAPD Fluid is Important in CAPD Patients

Benedik M[a], Ponikvar R[a], Guček A[a], Varl J[a], Buturović-Ponikvar J[a], Kveder R[a], Merc J[b]

[a]University Medical Center, Department of Nephrology, Ljubljana,

[b]Faculty of Pharmacy, Ljubljana, Slovenia

The concentrations of $25OHD_3$ and 1.25 $(OH)_2D_3$ in chronic renal failure patients are quite low.

The purpose of the study was to evaluate the serum concentrations of $25OHD_3$ and 1.25 $(OH)_2D_3$ in chronic hemodialysis (CHD) patients and in patients in CAPD program and to study the elimination of $25OHD_3$ and 1.25 $(OH)_2D_3$ with CAPD fluid During the first part of the study we measured serum concentration of $25OHD_3$ and 1.25$(OH)_2D_3$ in 42 CHD and in 45 CAPD patients. The concentrations of both forms of vitamin D were lower in CAPD patients. The results are in the table.

In the second part of the study we measured the elimination of 1.25 $(OH)_2D_3$ in CAPD fluid in 13 stable CAPD patients. Mean concentration of 1.25 $(OH)_2D_3$ in serum of these patients was 9.13 ± 7.97pmol/l, mean concentration in CAPD fluid measured in the morning before the next exchange was 6.32 ± 3.8pmol/l.

In the third part of the study we studied the elimination of vitamin D binding globuline (DBP) with CAPD fluid in 20 CAPD patients. Mean concentrations of serum DBP was 0.33g/l, mean concentration of DBP in CAPD fluid was 8.2mg/l.

For the determinations of concentrations of $25OHD_3$ and 1.25 $(OH)_2D_3$ RIA method was used. For the determinations of concentrations of DBP in CAPD fluid rocket immuno-electrophoresis (sec. Laurell) was used.

We can conclude that low serum concentrations of $25OHD_3$ and 1.25 $(OH)_2D_3$ in CAPD patients are on account of important elimination of vitamin D with CAPD fluid.

62

Prevalence of Anti-HCV Antibody in Chronic Hemodialysis Patients (Multi-Center Study)

H. Kim[a], K.T. Kim[a], Y.C. Chon[a], S.J. Lee[a], E.J. Lee[b], S.E. Park[c], S.Y. Suh[d], S.S. Kim[e], D.R. Cha[e], J.R. Koo[e], Y.J. Koo[e], Y.J. Kwon[e], W.Y. Cho[e], H.K. Kim[e]

Department of Internal Medicine[a], Koryo General Hospital, [b]Seoul Advantist Hospital, [c]Songnam Central Hospital, [d]Seoul Red Corss Hospital, [e]Korea University Hospital, Seoul, Korea

Purpose and Methods. We performed an epidemiological study of hepatitis C virus (HCV) infection on 224 patients of urban hemodialysis units to evaluate the prevalence and risk factors of HCV infection in patients with end stage renal disease on chronic hemodialysis.

Results. The male to female ratio and mean age were 116 cases vs 118 cases and 48 ± 14 years vs 50 ± 14 years. Using second generation RIA or ELISA test, the prevalence of anti HCV antibody were 14.7% (33 cases of 224 patients) and the mean duration and frequency of hemodialysis, amount of transfusion were significantly higher in anti HCV antibody positive group than negative group as follows (Duration of hemodialysis: 24 ± 17 months vs 17 ± 16 months, Frequency of hemodialysis: 634 ± 666 sessions vs 146 ± 156 sessions, Amount of transfusions: 13 ± 16 units vs 6 ± 9 units, $p < 0.05$). But there was no statistically significant difference in the sex ratio, mean age, level of AST and ALT, positivity of HBsAg between 2 groups.

Conclusion. From the above results, prevalence of HCV antibody in patients with hemodialysis has significant relation with hemodialysis duration and transfusion amount. It suggest that environmental factors of hemodialysis room and transfusion amount are major risk factors of HCV infection in patients with hemodialysis.

63

Endotoxin Level in Dialysis Systems

Sung K. Kang, Kyung S. Lee, Jae H. Kim, Jung K. Koh, Sung K. Park

Department of Medicine, Chonbuk National University, Medical School, Chonju, Korea

All bacterial cell walls contain peptidoglycan (PGG), Gram-negative bacteria contain an extra layer in the cell wall structure called the outer membrane, which is outside the PDG layer. Ecdotoxin (ET) is a component of this outer membrane. Endotoxin is generally a heat-stable toxin, has the various biological activities as pyrogenicity, macrophage & complement activation. The high performance membrane (HPM) dialyzers can remove large molecules like 10,000 MW ones in blood. In other words, 10,000 MW molecules in dialysis solutions can come into blood. Some dialysis patients are troubled with fever for unknown origin. It is assumed that pyrogens in dialysis solutions come into blood through dialyzers. A typical pyrogen is endotoxin. The condensed solutions are diluted with reverse osmosis (RO) water. Since the pore size of RO membrane is very small, endotoxin can be removed. The RO stored water is one of the source of endotoxin. Dialyzer inlet part connects tubing to dialyzer and is often contaminated with bacteria. So in order to protect the dialysis solution from bacterial & endotoxin contamination, we are proposed measures ET in the dialysis system by toxinometer (Limulus test, Wako) at 9 dialysis center in Korea. A RO system appeared necessary for decreasing ET in tap water to a certain concentration so ET in the dialysate would be minimal, as shown in figure.

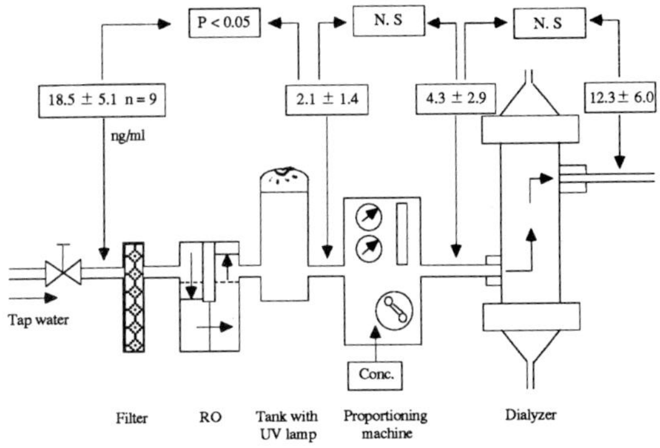

Table to Abstract 64

	FH 88	PAN 110	F 80	BLS 632	Filtral 20
Qb=200	25	26.1	20	20.6	19.5
Qb=300	24.4	24.5	18.8	20.3	19.3
Qb=400	24.5	23.5	18.3	21.6	18.6

64

Which Membrane for Predilution HF?

D. Hillion, T. Haas, C. Savoiu, A. Elbouatmani, M. Uzan, N. Pertuiset.

CHI Poissy and CMCO Evry, France

Large exchange volumes are needed to achieve high quality predilution HF (PreHF). We studied 5 different high flux high surface area membranes in terms of ultrafiltration rates to obtain guideline for the best choice in PreHF, between FH88 (Gambro Polyamide sqm), PAN 110 (Asahi PAN Dx 2.2 sqm), F 80 (Fresenius Polysulfone 1.8 sqm), BLS 632 (Sorin Polysulfone 1.8 sqm) and Filtral 20 (Hospal An69 2.0sqm). All membranes were used with Gambro AK100 Ultra at Qb = 200, 300 and 400ml/min and TMP ranging from 50 to 350mmHg. The table shows results for TMP = 300mmHg an a the graph the UF/TMP fluctuations for Qb = 400ml/min:

UF rate at Qb=400 ml/min

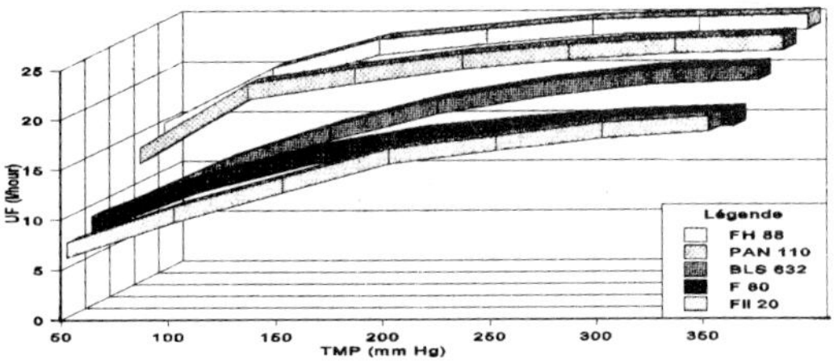

For all membranes increasing TMP above 300mmHg does not improve the UF rate (TMP independent Uf zone). Only PAN 110 and FH 88 are able to provide UF rate > 22*l*/h irrespective of the blood flow rate, allowing to exchange easily 60 to 70 liters in 3 hours at low transmembrane pressure. The other three membranes are unsuitable for use in predilution HF.

65

No Relationship between Increase in Extracoporeal Clearances and Small Molecules Mass Removal

T. Haas, D. Hillion, M J. Guerrito, M. Robine, M. Uzan, N. Pertuiset.

CMCM Evry and CHI Poissy, France

Increase in solute delayed mass transfer with increased extracorporeal clearances (ECC) during high efficiency sessions (HD or HDF) could be a limiting factor to further decrease in session time. We studied the influence of increasing ECC over plasma reduction rate (PRR) and total solute mass removal in two patients. Membrane = Fresenius F 80; Monitor = Gambro AK 100 Ultra. Each patient was treated on HDF one week at Qb = 200ml/min and RI = 50ml/min, one week at Qb = 300 and RI = 80 and one week at Qb = 400 and RI = 100. Whole blood clearances (Kb in ml/min) were calculated twice per session. Urea, Creatinine, Uric Acid and Phosphate were measured before and after session and QUANTISPAL (Hospal) was used to calculate total mass removal (TMR) in effluent dialysate. Paired Student's t-test was used for all values between each period. Results were as follows;

A 30% increase in ECC was observed between Qb = 200 and Qb = 300 and a further 20% between Qb = 300 and 400. There was no significant difference in presession plasma solutes levels between each period.

Except for creatinine from Qb = 200 to Qb = 300 there was no significant difference in TMR despite a significant increase in PRR for Urea, Creatinine and Uric Acid. For phosphate no significant difference was observed between low (142ml/min) and high (228ml/min) ECC, neither for PRR nor TMR.

These results argue against any increase in small molecules removal with increase in ECC and confirm the influence of delayed mass transfer in total solute removal during high flux EC treatment.

Table to Abstract 65

		Qb=200	t	Qb=300	t	Qb=400
Urea	PRR	75%	< 0.01	81%	< 0.01	84%
	Kb	183	< 0.001	258	< 0.001	317
mMol	TMR	497	NS	471	NS	495
Creat	PRR	66%	< 0.001	75%	< 0.01	79%
	Kb	147	< 0.001	215	< 0.001	271
μMol	TMR	14251	< 0.01	15872	NS	15003
U Acid	PRR	78%	< 0.01	86%	NS	87%
	Kb	159	< 0.001	223	< 0.001	280
	TMR	4950	NS	4947	NS	5307
Phos	PRR	48%	NS	50%	NS	46%
	Kb	142	< 0.01	189	< 0.01	228
mMol	TMR	18	NS	20	NS	20

66

Effect of Dialysate Composition on Coagulation and Thrombotic Parameters in Biofiltration

Taketoshi Hoshino[a], Jun-Ichi Onuki[a], Yukio Tsuruta[a], Takshi Shibamoto[b], Takashi Akiba[b].

[a]Yamato Hospital and [b]Kidney center, Tokyo Medical & Dental University, Tokyo, Japan

The biofiltration is a new treatment method for maintenance of end stage renal disease patients. One of the main problem is increment of filter coagulation accident during biofiltration. We hypothesed unphysiological pH of dialysates might affect coagulation activities. Study protocol were designed to address the effect of dialysate composition on coagulation and thrombotic parameters, *in vitro* and clinical.

Recirculation batch system was used study *in vitro*. Discarded plasma from immunological disease patient were used as blood substitute. Three different composition of dialysate such as acetate free biofiltration dialysate (AFD), acetate additional biofiltration dialysate (AAD) and conventional bicarbonate dialysate (CHD) were used. In clinical study, the substitution fluid were jutamin substitution (Fuso Pharma. Osaka, Japan) and bicarbonate substitutuion. Five patients were treated in this procedure. Coagulation and thrombotic parameters were thrombin antithrombin complex (TAT), pH, ionized calcium, fibrinopeptide A, alpha-2plasmin inhibitor complex (PIC), D-dimer, beta-thromboglobulin (BTG) and platelet factor-IV (PF4).

In *in vitro* study, the changes in TAT levels at 60 minute after contact with plasma and CHD, AFD and AAD were 14.2, 238 and 831 ng/ml. Increased TAT level in AAD were significantly larger than that with dialysates. The pH of CHD, AFD and AAD were 7.24 (CHD), 6.3 (AFD) and 6.2 (AAD), respectively. Ionized calcium levels were not significantly different among three dialysate. In clinical study, %changes of TAT levels were 72% (CHD), 25% (AFD) and 101% (AAD) when dialysate were not supplied. The increase in TAT with AAD was the highest level in three dialysates. Difference of % pH were not significant between CHD and AFD. The pH was the lowest level in AAD, among three dialysates. PIC, BTG and PF4 were not significantly different by dialysate composition.

AAD showed *in vitro* effects on coagulation parameters. AAF has less effect on coagulation parameters than those of the other dialysate in the clinical study. Lowered pH and/or acetate itself may play a part in filter coagulation accident. The changes of dialysate and substitution fluid composition might decrease these accident.

67

Efficacy of Hemodialysis to Eliminate Radiocontrast Material, Iohexol, soon after Angiography in Patients with Chronic Renal Failure

Naoto Sano, Hisato Sakamoto, Takashi Shibamoto, Teiichi Tamura, Takashi Akiba, Hiroshi Oshima, Fumiaki Marumo

Kinedy Center, Tokyo Medical and Dental University, Tokyo, Japan

Radiocontrast materials has adverse effect as a

nephrotoxin to induce acute renal dysfunction, especially in the patients with preexisting renal insufficiency. To eliminate the radiocontrast material by hemodialysis (HD) soon after angiography may reduce the nephrotoxity of this agent. In the present study, we examined the efficacy of HD to wash-out radiocontrast material in focus on the mechanism of elimination of this agent under both *in vivo* and *in vitro* conditions using almost same three kinds of dose material[iohexol (μg/ml) : low; 1,000, middle; 5,000, high; 15,000]. The study *in vitro* was done in a recirculating (5,000ml dialysate) batch system (QB 100ml/min, QD 500ml/min) for 2 hrs. On the other hand, *in vivo* study the serum concentration of iohexol was monitored before and after HD at 15, 30, 60, 90, 120min in 11 case (M/F; 6/5) with CRF (serum creatinine 2.0 - 7.0mg/dl). HD was performed using cellulose triacetate (CTA) membrane dialyzer in both studies. The serum iohexol concentration was monitored for 72 hr after administration. The concentration of iohexol was measured by HPLC. The reduction rate was maximum within 60min after HD (55$\pm$6% at 60min after HD), and 80 - 90% at 120min after HD in the presence of low or middle concentration of iohexol. But, in the presence of high dose iohexol the reduction rate was 55 - 60% at 120min even after HD. The clearance of iohexol was almost same as compared with that of creatinine (Ccm 82$\pm$5ml/min, Ccr 85$\pm$6ml/min). In addition, the possibility of adsorption of iohexol into dialyzer membrane was negligible. In all cases except for 2 cases, the serum creatinine concentration after angiography was returned to the basal level 48 hr later after HD.

Takentogether, these findings suggest that HD for 3 hr is effective to wash-out iohexol only at low and middle concentration. In contrast, at high dose concentration the adequate way to eliminate material from blood more effectively should be further examined.

68

Clinical Aspects of The AV Fistula Survival in Chronic Hemodialysis Patients (Multi-Center-Study)

Yong Seop Kim[a], Sun Sook Kim[a], Dae Ryong Cha[a], Won Yong Cho[a], Hyoung Kyu Kim[a], Eun Joo Lee[b], Hyang Kim[c], Sang Jong Lee[c], Sang Yeol Suh[d], Young Joo Kwon[e]

Department of Internal Medicine,
[a]Anam Hospital, Korea University,
[b]Seoul Adventist Hospital,
[c]Seoul Koryo Hospital,
[d]Seoul Red Cross Hospital,
[e]Kuro Hospital, Korea University

Purpose. Management of repeated long-term access to the vascular system is essential in care of patients with end stage renal disease (ESRD) treated with hemodialysis.

With aging dialysis population and increasing number of patients with peripheral vascular diseases such as diabetes mellitus, maintenance of adequate vascular access is clinically important. So we performed multicenter study for survival rate of AV fistula in chronic hemodialysis patients.

Method. We observed 9 parameters including underlying diseases, age, sex, site of AV fistula on 206 ESRD patients with hemodialysis from 6 hospitals for survival rate.

Results. (1) In 206 patients population, more than half (53%) were above 50 year old, and frequent underlying renal diseases were CGN (34.5%), diabetic nephropathy (25.2%), hypertensive nephropathy (18.4%). (2) Main type of AV fistula was radio-cephalic type (90.3%), end-to-side anastomosis (46%), and forearm (72%) was most frequent site of AV fistula. (3) Complications of AV fistula ware thrombosis (22 cases), aneurysm (5 cases), venous hypertension, infection, but incidence of thrombosis was higher significantly in older patients (4 times), in diabetic patients (5 times) ($p < 0.05$). (4) Average 1 year, 2 year and 3 year survival rates of AV fistulas in total population were 86.5%, 83.0%, 79.5%, and the mean survival period was 38.2 months. Mean survival rate of AV fistulas in older patients was lower significantly than in younger patients($p < 0.05$). (5) Comparing to non-diabetic patients, 1 year, 2 year and 3 year survival rates of AV fistulas in diabetic patients were lower significantly ($p < 0.05$)

But, type & site of AV fistula, mode of anastomosis,

specialty of operator, sex of patients were not correlated with fistula survival.

Conclusion. AV fistula survival rate was significantly lower in diabetic patients and old patients, so we should manage AV fistula more carefully to prevent thrombosis in old & diabetic ESRD patients with hemodialysis.

69

Effects of Dialysis Membranes on Platelet Aggregation

YJ Kwon, NH Kim, MK Chang, YH Lee, YS Kim, DR Cha, WY Cho, HJ PYO, HK Kim

Department of Internal Medicine, Korea University, Seoul, Korea

Clinically significant interactions between blood & dialysis membranes occur during hemodialysis. Platelet interactions with dialysis membranes have been observed such as decrease in platelet count, platelet adhesiveness & retention to dialysis membranes, platelet degranulation &formation of platelet microaggregates. Marked defects in platelet functions, such as their aggregation response were also noted to be present following dialysis. To evaluate the biocompatibility of different dialysis membranes (cuprophane & polymethylethacrylate (PMMA)) by platelet aggregation, we measured platelet aggregation to ADP, epinephrine, collagen, ristocetin before and after dialysis in 7 chronic hemodialysis patients (M:F = 4:3, mean age: 51.4 ± 12.0 years).

Methods. Each patient underwent dialysis for 6 wks with 2 dialyzer under same conditions. Blood samples were taken at the pre- & post dialysis before switching to the other type of dialyzer. The sequence of dialyzer was cuprophane, followed by PMMA dialyzer.

Results. (1) Platelet aggregation to ADP, epinephrine was increased after HD of each dialysis membrane. (ADP-cuprophane vs. PMMA: 17.2 ± 11.0 vs, 4.9 ± 14.2, $p > 0.05$, epinephrine-cuprophane vs. PMMA: 18.6 ± 20.4 vs. 10.3 ± 12.2, $p > 0.05$). (2) Platelet aggregation to collagen, ristocetin was increased after HD of cuprophane dialysis membrane, but decreased after HD of PMMA membrane. (collagen-cuprophane vs. PMMA: 6.8 ± 28.4 vs. -4.6 ± 7.8, $p > 0.05$, ristocetin-cuprophane vs. PMMA: 28.4 ± 26.2 vs. -9.0 ± 12.1, $p > 0.05$).

Conclusion. PMMA membrane may also cause platelet dyfunction during hemodialysis.

70

Role of Cytokines in Malnutrition

Charles A. Dinarello

Tufts University and New England Medical Center, Boston, MA USA

Accelerated loss of body cell mass (BCM) is characteristic of patients with trauma, infections and chronic inflammatory diseases. The cytokines interleukin-1 (IL-1) and tumor necrosis factor (TNF) have been linked to the pathogenesis of cachexia and wasting since infusions of these cytokines either alone or together onto animals results in anorexia and loss of BCM.

Controversy arose when some studies showed that incubating muscle tissue in vitro with IL-1, TNF or a 5,000 mol wt serum factor induced proteolysis whereas other studies showed no effect. However, in rats injected with IL-1, ex vivo muscle proteolysis with increased myofibrillar protein has been reported. The IL-1-induced proteolysis was not mediated by endogenous glucocorticoids. Moreover, in rats made septic following cecal ligation and puncture, blocking IL-1 receptors with a constant infusion of IL-1 receptor antagonist normalized the increased rate of muscle protein breakdown. Anorexia induced by IL-1 or TNF animals during an inflammatory reaction reduces weight loss and anorexia. The reduction in anorexia is thought to be due to a decrease in IL-1 and TNF-induced IL-6 release. In humans, a positive correlation ($p < 0.001$) has been made with the cellular production of TNF and IL-1β and the resting energy expenditure. Patients with chronic inflammation (rheumatoid arthritis) have a 13% lower BCM ($p < 0.00001$) than age, sex and weight matched control subjects. Energy intake in these patients is inversely correlated with production of IL-1β ($p < 0.005$). It is concluded that cytokines such as IL-1 and TNF directly stimulate muscle breakdown and induce the anoretic cytokine IL-6; together, both processes result in cachexia and wasting.

71

The Survival Rate and Causes of Death in Patients with Chronic Renal Failure on Hemodialysis

Kyoung Won Kahng, Jeong Ho Kim, Ji Hoon Kim, Ho Jung Kim, Chan Hyun Park, Chong Myung Kang, Han Chul Park

Department of Internal Medicine, College of Medicine, Hangyang University, Sooul, Korea

Purpose. Regular hemodialysis had been established as a way of treatment for end stage renal failure. There are many reports on long term follow-up for chronic hemodialysis patients. We analyzed the patients with chronic renal failure on hemodialysis.

Method. In a retrospective study, the survival rate and the causes of death were analyzed in 548 patients with chronic renal failure on hemodialysis during the period of 1982 to 1991, treated at the Hanyang University Hospital. The patients were mostly dialysed 2 to 3 times a week for 4 to 5 hours.

Results. The demographic characteristics of these patients, male to female ratio was 58:42 and the mean age was 47.2 ± 13.7 years. Underlying disorders of chronic renal failure consisted of mainly chronic glomerulonephritis (23.5%). followed by diabetic nephropathy (15.9%), and hypertensive nephrosclerosis (13.9%). The causes of death were most frequently cerebrovascular accidents (25.9%), including hemorrhage and infarction, followed by cardiac disorders (19.4%), infections (16.7%), and gastrointestinal bleedings (6.5%). The overall of survival rates in hemodialysis patients were 85.6% for 1 year, 75.3% for 2 year, 62.3% for 5 years, 33.7% for 10 years. Dividing into subgroups, renal failure due to diabetes and hypertensive nephrosclerosis carried significantly poor outcomes. The survival rate of the older patients were shorter than the younger patients ($p < 0.001$).

Conclusion. We should pay attention to the hemodialysis patients during the first year because survival rate of this period was shorter than other period.

72

The correlation between the Kinetic Indices and Rehabilitation in the Patients on Maintenance Hemodialysis

Kyoung Won Kahng, Jeong Ho Kim, Ji Hoon Kim, Ho Jung Kim, Chan Hyun Park, Chong Myung Kang, Han Chul Park

Department of Internal Medicine, College of Medicine, Hanyang University, Seoul, Korea

Purpose. The urea kinetic modeling has been used as useful index for adequate dialysis in hemodialysis patients. We performed this study to evaluate the usefulness of kinetic index for degree of rehabilitation.

Method. The kinetic indices using urea kinetic modeling and degree of rehabilitation were analysed 105 patients with chronic renal failure on hemodialysis treated at the Hanyang University Hospital.

Results. The dermographic characteristics of these patients, male to female was 58:42 and the mean age was 46.8 ± 12.7 years. Underlying disorders of chronic renal nephrosclerosis (14.3%). and diabetic nephropathy (7.6%). Family status was significant in that 18 cases (58%) were married and 32.3% (10) were never married, the remaining 3 (9.7%) were divorced or widowed. Of the total 105 patients, 31 (43.1%) are presently employed. Of those 31 working patients, 16 were selfemployed, 8 were on service jobs and 3 were on general office jobs. More than half (63.1%) of those patients worked full-time, 9 (29%) part-time, and 3 (9.7%) irregularly. Only 72 (68.6%) patients held jobs before dialysis, and 16 (22.2%) of those returned to the same job. The physical activity of the patients were statistically not related with urea kinetic indices such as PCR, Kt/V, total KT/V/week, TACurea, nor with hematocrit ($p > 0.05$). However, in serum albumin level the difference between group 0, 1, 2 and group 3, 4 in physical activity was significant ($p < 0.05$). The patients dialysed below 2 times per week had lower values of Kt/V, total KT/V/wk, and PCR than the patients dialysed more than 2 times per week ($p < 0.01$).

Conclusion. From the above results, it appeared that kinetic indices using urea kinetic modeling are not closely related to the degree of rehabilitation in hemodialysis patients.

73

Assessment of Nutrition in Dialysis Patients

Peter G Kerr

Department of Nephrology, Monash Medical Center, Clayton, 3168. Australia

The assessment of nutritional status in dialysis patients has gained in importance as clinicians have realized the close correlation that exists between nutritional status and long term outcome. The question remains, however, as to how nutrition is best assessed in this group. Much reliance in recent years has been placed on the use of urea kinetics, both in the assessment of dialysis adequacy and for estimating the protein catabolic rate (PCR), the latter as an index of nutrition. Many are sceptical of the interdependence of these values and their subsequent correlation. In addition, calculation of the PCR relies on the assumption that the patient is not catabolic (or anabolic) at the time of measurement a common circumstance in ill patients. Alternative indices of nutrition that have been utilized frequently include anthropometric measurements such as height, weight, skin-fold thickness and arm circumference as well as the body-mass index. These indices are relatively insensitive to changes in nutritional status and norms vary considerably between racial groups.

This may be a considerable problem in cosmopolitan societies. Biochemical markers such as serum albumin and prealbumin, and transferrin have also been widely used. Correlations have been drawn between albumin levels and survival in dialysis patients, however, the applicability of these results to individual patients is questionable (as opposed to population studies). Other biochemical markers such as IGF-1 have yet to be fully explored. Gold standard techniques for assessment of body composition can be helpful but are often cumbersome for routine clinical use. In-vivo neutron activation analysis for assessment of total body nitrogen for example is felt to be very accurate and reproducible but is available to only a few renal units. On the other hand, the emergence of techniques such as bio-electrical impedance and DEXA has made assessment of body water, fat mass, and fat-free mass more easily available. Although the accuracy of these techniques may not be as great as multi-compartment models of body composition, their ease of clinical application makes them attractive. Data is only beginning to emerge on the usefulness of these techniques for nutritional assessment in dialysis patients although they have been well validated in normals and have already been used extensively for volume assessment in dialysis patients.

Refinement of these techniques may provide significant, reproducible nutritional information about our dialysis patients.

74

Elevated Serum C-Reactive Protein (CRP) is a Strong Predictor of Increased Mortality and Low Serum Albumin in Hemodialysis (HD) Patients

Bergström J, Heimbürger O, Lindholm B, Qureshi AR

Division of Renal Medicine and Baxter Novum, Karolinska Institite, Huddinge, Sweden

Several reports demonstrate that low serum albumin (A) levels are associated with increased risk of death in HD patients. It is therefore generally assumed that malnutrition is a strong risk factor for increased mortality. However, A is also influenced by non-nutritional factors such as age, overhydration, increased capillary permeability and inflammatory conditions; A is a "negative" acute phase protein (APP). An APP response is commonly recorded as an increase in CRP. We evaluated nutritional status in 128 HD patients (M/F 76/52, age 61 ± 14 y) by subjective global assessment (SGA) and measured several anthropometric and biochemical nutrition markers and also measured CRP. All measurements were made on a non-dialysis day after an overnight fast. The patients were then followed for 4 years and mortality was analyzed in relation to SGA, A, CRP

Table to Abstract 74

Survival	sAlbumin g/L			sCRP mg/L		
	> 35 n = 33	30-35 n = 69	< 30 n = 16	< 15 n = 81	15-30 n = 23	> 30 n = 23
1 year	83%	79%	56%	95%	80%	46%
3 year	69%	48%	0%	72%	38%	22%

and several other factors (Kaplan-Meyer, log-rank tests, multiple regression). SGA and A and CRP all predicted survival.

The table shows that CRP appeared to be a better predictor of 1-y survival than A and as good a predictor of 3-y survival as A. CRP and A were inversely correlated ($r = -0.33$, $p < 0.001$) supporting that A behaves as a "negative" APP. Multiple regression demonstrates CRP to be a stronger predictor ($p < 0.004$) than SGA ($p < 0.001$) of A. This suggests that non-nutritional factors (inflammation, infection, tissue injury) resulting in increased APP production are at least as influential on A as the nutritional stage; such factors seem to have an important role for the clinical outcome as demonstrated by our results.

75

Loss of Ultrafiltration in Continuous Ambulatory Peritoneal Dialysis (CAPD) -A 15 Year Study

Olof Heimbürger, Jacek Waniewski, Andrzej Werynski, Anders Trasnæus, Bengt Lindholm

Karolinska Institute, Stockholm, Sweden and Institute of Biocybernetics and Biological Engineering, Warsaw, Poland

Permanent loss of ultrafiltration capacity (UFC) is a wellknown complication during long term CAPD treatment. The most common mechanism for loss of UFC is rapid glucose absorption (RGA) and thus rapid loss of the osmotic driving force whereas other mechanisms such as loss of peritoneal surface area with slow solute transport (SST) due to fibrosis and the formation of adhesions or increased peritoneal fluid absorption (IFA) also have been reported.

The aim of the present study was to evaluate the incidence and the different mechanisms for UFC in our total adult CAPD population during a 15 year period.

Loss of UFC was defined as: edema and inability to reach "dry weight" despite three or more hypertonic exchanges (3.86%) per day and a restricted fluid intake with duration of symptoms of overhydration > 1 month, and no established cause of UFC loss such as peritonitis, dialysate leakage or catheter malfunction. The mechanism of UFD loss was evaluated using the peritoneal equilibration test (PET) or using a six hour dwell study with ^{131}I-radioiodinated albumin (RISA) as a volume marker. In the dwell studies, the total fluid absorption rate was estimated by the disappearance rate (K_E, ml/min) of RISA from the peritoneal cavity and lymphatic absorption was estimated by the rate of RISA appearance in plasma.

During the period 1978-1993, 22 out of 365 adult patients trained for CAPD at out unit developed loss of UFC; 20/22 of these patients were studied.

One patients studied with PET showed low UFC and normal solute transport which may be due to IFA or reduced ultrafiltration coefficient. Lymphatic absorption was below 20% of the total peritoneal fluid absorption rate in all studied patients ($n = 12$) irrespective of the mechanism of UFC.

We conclude that (1) loss of UFC is afflicting about 6% of CAPD patients, (2) increased peritoneal fluid absorption is a rare cause of UFC loss, accounting for only about 25% of the cases of UFC loss, and that (3) increased lymphatic absorption does not seem to play any major role in UFC loss.

76

On-Line HDF-A Safe and Efficient Way to Increase β_2m Removal

T. Shinzato[a], M. Miwa[a], S. Nakai[a], M. Takahashi[b], S. Tsutsui[b], M. Ono[c], H. Ogawa[c], K. Maeda[a]

[a]Nagoya univ. branch hospital internal medicine,
[b]Aoi central hospital
[c]Shinseikai daiichi hospital

This study was designed to show that on-line hemodiafiltration (OHDF) is a safe method to increase the removal of β_2-microglobulin (β_2m). For each of 7 male and 3 female patients from 2 centers (group A) one month of normal hemodialysis (HD) was followed by one month of OHDF. Also, 4 additional patients were

Table to Abstract 75

	RGA	SST	IFA
PET (n = 8)	7/8 (87.5%)	0	not determinded
Dwell study (n = 12)	9*/12 (75%)	0	4*/12 (30%)

* including a combined pattern (RGA+IFA) in one patient

followed for 3 months on OHDF (group B). All patients had previously been on bicarbonate HD. Blood flow (200-250ml/min), treatment time (4-5 hours) and dialyzer type (1.6m^2 polyamide, Gambro AB) were kept unchanged for each patient during the entire study. Samples for analysis of β_2m and urea were obtained from the fistula needle pre and post treatment following the long dialysis free interval of the week, and were drawn before connection and after disconnection to the extracorporeal circuit. RIA- (Sionogi) or Latex enzyme agglutination (LX-EIKEN) technique was used to analyze β_2m, and post treatment values were corrected for extracellular volume change according to Bergström. Urea was analyzed using standard laboratory equipment (Hitachi 7350), and KT/V was calculated. Dialysis fluid was perpared from liquid A-concentrate (AF-2, Kindaly) and dry bicarbonate powder (BiCart, Gambro AB) and was checked for fluid composition once every week using standard laboratory methods. Samples for microbiological evaluation of the fluid were collected every second week from 6 positions along the fluid path, and the final fluid was checked every week. The chromogenic limulus test Toxicolor system (Seikagaku Kogyo CO LTD, Japan) was used for endotoxin analysis, and Tryptone Glucose Extract Agar was used for bacteria culturing for 7 days at 25℃. The fluid composition was found to be in perfect agreemint with expectations with an excellent microbiological quality. Except for the incoming water, all endotoxin values were below the limit 0.01EU/ml, and no bacteria were found in the final fluid. As expected there was no change in hemoglobin, erythrocytes, leucocytes, thrombocytes, hematocrit, Na^+, K^+, Ca^{2+}, urea, creatinine, phosphate, bicarbonate, pCO2, pH, total protein, albumin, GOT or GPT during the study, and no change in blood pressure, heart rate or body temperature during the treatments. OHDF exchange volumes per treatment were 20.2±1.6 l in group A, and 21.8±3.1 l in group B. The percent reduction in β_2m and KT/V for urea were as shown in table

As expected there is a significant in β_2m reduction by OHDF, which persistent over longer time, but only a slight increase in KT/V. The relatively high removal in HD is due to the use of a high flux membrane in combination with long treatments (> 4hrs) and small patients. There was a surprisingly large difference in KT/V between the two clinics. This was due to a large difference in patient weight, which was not fully compensated by choice of treatment parameters. The efficiency and safety of OHDF for increased removal of β_2m is thus supported.

77

Synergic Effects of ET and PG on Production of Cytokine in Mononuclear Cells of Renal Failure Patients

Kenji Tsuchida[a], Yoshiaki Takemoto[a], Seiji Yamagami[a], Taketoshi Kishimoto[a], Makoto Niwa[a], Stanley Shaldon[b]

[a]Osaka City University
[b]University Hospital Nimes

Purpose. We proved the existence of peptidoglycan (PG) in dialysate using Silkworm Larvae Plasma (SLP) reagent. Since dialysate is contaminated with PG, there is a possibility that PG interferes with the biological reactions in ET-contaminated dialysate. Therefore, in order to clarify the clinical significance of PG, we studied biological activation in dialysate where PG exists alone and where ET and PG coexist.

Method. We studied the effect of Peripheral Blood Mononuclear Cells (PBMC) of healthy controls on production of cytokine (IL-1RA, IL-1) in vitro using LPS of E. coli as ET, Muramyl dipeptide (MDP) as a fragment of PG and contaminant dialysate. Furthermore a comparative study was made of the synergic effect of ET and MDP on cytokine renal failure.

Results and Conclusion. In healthy controls, cytokine production of PBMC was synergically effected by MDP and ET. Similar results were also obtained after adding contaminant dialysate. Synergic effects of ET and MDP were lower in PBMC of CAPD and HD patients compared with healthy controls. The effects were significantly lower among patients receiving contaminant dialysate and HPM in HD group and were proportional to the length of treatment. Therefore, in HD group there is a possibility of pyrogen influx in the course of the treatment. A mechanism of increasing tolerance for ET and PG may also develop in the patients.

Table to Abstract 76

	HD	OHDF	p	OHDF group B
% red. β_2-M	59±7	76±10	< 0.01 (n = 40)	79±5
KT/V urea	1.57±0.25	1.61±0.25	< 0.05 (n = 40)	1.62±0.36

Table to Abstract 79

	Calcium 1.25		Calcium 1.75		1.25 vs 1.75
	pre	post	pre	post	p
i-Ca	1.13 (0.15)	1.11 (0.11)	1.13 (0.16)	1.33 (0.15)[a]	< 0.001
SBP	139 (20)	121 (18)[a]	140 (26)	135 (19)	0.010
DBP	82 (12)	77 (13)	81 (12)	82 (11)	0.022
MAP	105 (16)	96 (18)[b]	105 (19)	105 (16)	0.021
HR	69 (7)	79 (10)[a]	69 (10)	77 (13)[a]	NS
FVR	1626 (729)	2480 (1205)[a]	1555 (826)	2365 (1226)[b]	NS
VT	16.9 (4.6)	14.7 (5.0)[b]	16.6 (4.5)	14.3 (4.0)[b]	NS

mean (SD) ; post vs pre : [a] = $p < 0.01$, [b] = $p < 0.05$

78

Effects of Different Ultrafiltration Rates on Hemodynamic Parameters in Cardiac Compromised Patients (CCpts) and Patients with a normal Cardiac Function (NCpts)

F.M. van der Sande[a], A.W. Mulder[b], W.H.M. van Kuijk[a], K.M.L. Leunissen[a]

Department of Internal Medicine, [a]University Hospital Maastricht, Masstricht and [b]Catharina Hospital, Eindhoven, The Netherlands

The increasing number of elderly patients and patients with cardiovascular disease has the potential of an increase in the incidence of intradialytic hypotension. Intradialytic hypotension is determined by a decrease in plasma volume (PV) (dependent of UF-rate), the patient's cardiovascular status (decreased LV-compliance) and the treatment mode (influencing cardiovascular regulatory mechanisms).

Trerefore, we studied the influence of different UF-rates (500+1000ml/hr) on blood pressure (mmHg, Dynamap), PV (%, Hct-method), and interstitial volume (Res = resistivity units, BIA) during 2 hours combined UF+HD and 2 hours UF-only in 8 CCpts (ejection fraction < 35%) and 7 NCpts (ejection fraction > 35%). Dialysis was standardized: individual Bicarbonate; Sodium 141 mmol/l; Calcium 1.75 mmol/l; AN-'69 dialyzer. The changes from baseline are expressed as mean (SD) ; statistical analysis: repeated measurements MANOVA.

There were no significant differences between CCpts and NCpts. UF-only resulted in minor hemodynamic changes in both CCpts and NCpts. UF+HD resulted in a significant decrease in SBP at both UF-rates in CCpts while in contrast SBP decreased sgnificantly only during UF+HD-1000 in NCpts. The decrease in PV and increase in Res (= decrease of interstitial volume) was comparable between CCpts and NCpts and was only dependent on the UF-rate.

We conclude that differences in hemodynamic stability during UF+HD between CCpts and NCpts are not related to differences in PV-preservation. In addition, lower UF-rates should be advocated in CCpts during UF+HD.

Table to Abstract 78

	CCpts				NCpts			
	UF 500	UF 1000	UF+HD 500	UF+HD 1000	UF 500	UF 1000	UF+HD 500	UF+HD 1000
SBP	+4 (19)	-4 (22)	-11 (13)[a]	-27 (26)[bd]	+12 (7)[b]	-5 (16)	+4 (21)	-16 (10)[be]
DBP	+4 (9)	-1 (11)	-4 (9)	-5 (22)	+8 (9)[a]	+2 (7)	+3 (7)	-2 (10)
MAP	+5 (12)	-3 (16)	-2 (12)	-10 (24)	+7 (9)[a]	-1 (11)	+3 (13)	-7 (8)[e]
HR	-3 (8)	+4 (7)[c]	+2 (6)	+3 (9)	-2 (5)	-3 (6)	+1 (10)	+7 (6)[bd]
PV	-12 (3)[b]	-20 (7)[bc]	-9 (3)[b]	-17 (4)[be]	-8 (5)[b]	-20 (8)[bc]	-5 (6)[b]	-19 (8)[be]
Res	+28 (7)[b]	+50 (15)[bcd]	+23 (17)[b]	+42 (16)[be]	+24 (13)[b]	+45 (10)[b]	+19 (9)[b]	+40 (9)[be]

changes from baseline : [a] = $p < 0.05$ [b] = $p < 0.01$. changes between treatments within groups : UF-500 vs UF-1000, [c] = $p < 0.05$. UF-1000 vs UF+HD-1000, [d] = $p < 0.05$. UF+HD-500 vs UF+HD-1000, [e] = $p < 0.05$

79

The Effect of Changes in Plasma Ionized Calcium (i-Ca) on Blood Pressure and Vascular Reactivity during UF+HD

W.H.M van Kuijk[a], *A.W. Mulder*[b], *G.A. Harff*[c], *K.M.L. Leunissen*[a]

[a]Department of Internal Medicine, University Hospital Maastricht, Maastricht; Department of [b]Internal Medicine and [c]Clinical Chemistry, Catharina Hospital, Eindlhoven, The Netherlands

In order to prevent hypercalcaemia due to the treatment of secondary hyperparathyroidism it is advocated to use low calcium dialysate. However calcium ions play a pivotal role in myocardial contractility and could theoretically play a role in vascular smooth muscle contraction. Therefore, we studied the influence of changes in plasma i-Ca (mmol/l) on both vascular reactivity and blood pressure during dialysis in cardiovascular stable patients.

Changes in forearm vascular resistance (FVR; mmHg/ml/100ml/sec) and venous tone (VT; mmHg/ml/100ml) (strain-gauge plethysmography) as well as blood pressure (SBP, DBP, MAP; mmHg) and heart rate (HR; beats/min) were measured in 10 HD patients during two dialysis treatment that only differed in the dialysate calcium concentration; 1.25 and 1.75mmol/l. Dialysis; 3 hrs, Bicarbonate 34mmol/l, Sodium 140mmol/l, hemophane membranes (GFS-16, Gambro), UF-rate 0.80*l*/hr.

i-Ca was significantly higher during high Ca UF+HD, during which it increased significantly. All three blood pressure parameters were significantly lower during low Ca UF+HD: both SBP and MAP decreased significantly only during low Ca UF+HD. Vascular reactivity was comparable between the two treatments; FVR increased significantly while VT decreased significantly.

We conclude that changes in i-Ca are a very important determinant of the blood pressure response during UF+HD. However, vascular reactivity during UF+HD is not directly influenced by changes in i-Ca. These results suggest that the influence of changes in i-Ca on blood pressure is primary mediated by changes in myocardial contractility.

80

Viral Hepatitis in Dialysis Patients. Hepatitis C Viral Infection: Epidemiology

Jose M Morales

Hospital 12 de Octubre, Madrid, Spain

It is well known that non-A non-B hepatitis is a frequent complication in patients on chronic hemodialysis. Recently it has been demonstrated that hepatitis C virus (HCV) is responsible for 80-90% of non-A non-B hepatitis in dialysis patients. Prevalence of HCV infection (antibodies anti-HCV positive by ELISA2, RIBA2) in these patients varies widely (10-60%) among dialysis units of different countries. This variation is due to several factors, mainly the past transfusional policy of the unit. HCV infection in these patients is chronic in 90% of cases, showing that serum HCV RNA is the most useful marker of true infection and serum transaminase have low sensitivity to detect ongoing HCV. In general, the principal risk factors to acquire HCV infection in dialysis are: the number of transfusions, the duration on dialysis, previous renal transplant and the presence of antiHb core. Nevertheless, about 10% of patients with antibodies HCV positive had never been transfused. In this way, there are convincing data implicating nosocomial transmission of HCV within the dialysis setting. Until a vaccine becomes available and the usefulness of Interferon or Ribavirin as antiviral therapy is demonstrated, HCV prophylaxis should include to avoid transfusions and to eradicate of nosocomial infection. Changes in the recommendations for control of non-A non-B hepatitis in patients in chronic hemodialysis could be the main preventive measure for HCV infection.

81

Intermittent Venovenous Hemofiltration for The Treatment of Refractory Edema

H.C. Kim, I. Joo, J. Suk, S.B. Park

Division of Nephrology, Keimyung University School of Medicine, Taegu, Korea

Recently, continuous venovenous hemofiltration (CVVH) has been used an effective treatment of refractory edema. However, continued production of large ultrafiltrates during CVVH frequently results in life-threatening hypotension, which may prevent an adequate treatment. This problem can be improved when the CVVH is repeated intermittently at one or two days interval (IVVH). We compared CVVH and IVVH in the treatment of 50 patients with refractory edema. Although the mean duration of treatment was significantly longer in the CVVH (CVVH: 41±23 h, IVVH: 18±9 h; $p < 0.001$), the total ultrafilltration rate (UFR) was not significantly different between the two groups. The UFR per hour was 3 times higher in the IVVH groups (IVVH : 1.681±495ml, CVVH : 581± 323ml; $p < 0.001$). Net fluid removal was not significantly different between the two groups. Abdominal girth has decreased significantly in both groups, however, the percent decrement was greater in IVVH group (11% vs 7.8%). Changes in blood chemistry and hemodynamics before and after treatment were comparable in both groups. The incidence of hypotension during treatment was significantly lower in the IVVH group (IVVH: 20%, CVVH: 44% $p < 0.05$), and the rate of filter clotting was also significantly lower in the IVVH group (IVVH: 0%, CVVH: 48%, $p < 0.01$). The higher UFR per hour and the lower complication rate suggest that IVVH may be the preferred modality for patients with refractory edema.

82

Effect of Hemodialysis on Malondialdehyde and Antioxidnat Enzymes of Erythrocytes in Patients with Chronic Renal Failure

K.C Mun[a], C.S Kwak[a], I. Joo[b], S.B Park[b], H.C Kim[b]

[b]Department of Internal Medicine and [a]Biochemistry, Keimyung University School of Medicine, Taegu, Korea

Level of malondialdehyde (MDA) which is the lipid peroxidation product, and the activities of antioxidant enzymes such as superoxide dismutase (SOD), catalase, and glutathione peroxidase (GSH-Rx) were determined before and after hemodialysis in the erythrocytes (RBCs) from 20 patients with chronic renal failure (CRF), and from 14 healthy subjects to clarify the mechanism of the protective effect of hemodialysis on lipid peroxidation in RBC membrane structures. The amount of MDA was measured by the method of thiobarbituturic acid assay. Superoxide dismutase was assayed by the method of Hyland et al. Glutathione peroxidase activity was assayed by the method of Palgia and Valentine. Catalase activity was assayed by the method of Bregmyer. Before dialysis, MDA level (0.50±0.17 nmol MDA/mg protein in RBC, $p < 0.05$) and GSH-Px activity (42.49±7.93 nmol NADPH reduced/mg protein in RBC/min, $p < 0.001$) in chronic uremic patients were higher than those in healthy controls (0.38±0.08, and 17.71±8.81), while SOD(5.39±4.57 unit/mg protein in RBC/min, $p < 0.05$) and catalse (23.11±1.82 μmol H_2O_2 destroyed/mg protein in RBC/min, $p < 0.001$) activites were lower than those in healthy controls (8.59 ±3.09, and 31.20±3.26). This result suggested that enzymatic antioxidant defense mechanisms except GSH-Px are suppressed, and lipid peroxidation is increased in the RBCs from the patients with CRF. It means that reduced antioxidant defense mechanism in the RBSc is one of the factors leading to peroxidation in the lipid structure of the RBC membrane and thereby to hemolysis and anemia in the patients with CRF. After hemodialysis, MDA (0.41±0.08, $p < 0.05$ vs. predialysis), SOD (8.36±6.44, $p < 0.05$ vs. predialysis) and catalase (24.75±2.15, $p < 0.01$ vs. predialysis) in the RBCs from the patients with CRF were normalized, while GSH-Px (42.70±7.45) did not change. This result indicates that hemodialysis is helpful to protect the peroxidative damage through normalizing SOD and catalase activities in the RBCs.

83

Changes of Insulin-Like Growth Factor Binding Proteins (IGFBPs) in Patients on Maintenance Hemodialysis (HD)

Sung Kwang Park, Sung Kyew Kang, Dae-Yeol Lee

Department of Internal Medicine and Pediatrics, Chonbuk National University Medical School, Chonju, Korea

Insulin-like growth factor (IGF) -I & -II play essential roles in the modulation of cellular growth and differentiation and circulate in high concentration bound to several high affinity binding proteins (IGFBPs). The alteration of serum IGFs and IGFBPs have been reported in patients with acute and chronic renal failure. The current study sought to identify changes of serum IGFBPs profile in patients on maintenance HD. In this study, we measured IGFBPs by using western ligand blot (WLB) in the serum of 18 patients on maintenance HD and 6 control subject and analysed by densitometry.

Results showed (mean ± S.E; *, $p < 0.001$ after HD vs before HD) :

	before HD	after HD
IGFBP-1 (ADU)	0.40 ± 0.05	0.42 ± 0.07
IGFBP-2 (ADU)	2.61 ± 0.45	3.30 ± 0.54
IGFBP-3 (ADU)	10.18 ± 1.11	14.30 ± 1.50*
IGFBP-4 (ADU)	0.31 ± 0.04	0.35 ± 0.04

Mean serum IGFBP-3 level was 10.18 ± 1.11 (ADU) and increased to 14.30 ± 1.50 (ADU) after HD. Most patients on maintenance HD showed increased serum IGFBP-3, the most abundant serum IGFBP without any changes of IGFBP-1, -2 and -4.

We speculate that increase in serum IGFBP-3 profile during HD would be due to the alteration of some regulatory mechanisms of IGFBP-3 synthesis and these changes may contribute in part to hormonal and metabolic changes during HD.

84

Serum Soluble HLA Class I Antigen Levels in Hemodialysis Patients

CW Yang[a], TK Kim[b], YS Kim[a], WS Koo[a], H Han[b], EJ Choi[a], YS Chang[a], BK Bang[a]

[a]Department of Internal Medicine, [b]Department of Microbiology, Catholic University Medical College, Seoul, Korea

Uremia is characterized by preactivated immune state because the interaction of a blood-artificial membrane during hemodialysis (HD) procedure stimulates lymphocytes to produce cytokines that modulate the immune reaction. We measured the serum levels of soluble HLA class I antigen (sHLA-I) to evaluate the immune status of uremia. Twenty-one HD patients had serum samples collected for sHLA-I analysis before and after HD. The serum sHLA-I levels in patients undergoing HD were higher than in the normal controls (574.8 ± 431.1 vs. 415.6 ± 256.1 ng/ml, $p < 0.05$). HD duration was not correlated with serum sHLA-I levels ($r = 0.01$, $P > 0.05$), and pre- and post-HD serum sHLA-I levels were not significantly different (574.8 ± 431.1 vs. 568.3 ± 398.4 ng/ml, $P > 0.05$). In conclusion, elevated serum sHIA levels in a uremic status are more likely to be associated with metabolic derangement of sHLA-I rather than an immunologic reaction of lymphocytes by dialysis. This finding also suggests possibilities that lymphocyte stimulation by dialysis itself is not enough to release sHLA-l and the mechanism for releasing sHLA-I is different from cytokines.

85

Prevalence, Incidence and Risk Factors of Hepatitis C Virus Infection in Hemodialysis Patients: Multi-Center Study in Catholic Medical Center

SH Lee, CW Yang, SA Yoon, DC Jin, SJ Ahn, SY Kim, WS Koo, EJ Choi, YS Yoon, YS Chang, BK Bang

Department of Internal Medicine, Catholic University Medical College, Seoul Korea

This study was performed to evaluate the prevalence and incidence of hepatitits C virus (HCV) infection in patients undergoing hemodialysis (HD). 5 HD centers in catholic medical center were included. The prevalence of anti-HCV Ab in HD patients was 23.2% (36/155) at 1992, 21.7% (60/227) at 1993 and 22.2% (55/248) at 1994. The incidence of anti-HCV Ab was 9.3% (16/192) at 1993 and 5.2% (12/599) at 1994. Between the patients with positive conversion ($n = 28$) and without conversion ($n = 193$) of anti-HCV Ab, there were no differences in sex ratio, age, transfusion (unit/month) and proportion of diabetics. But, HD duration in patients with positive conversion was significantly longer than patients without conversion (50 ± 33 vs. 38 ± 28, $p < 0.05$) and elevation of transaminase was more frequently observed in patients with positive conversion (32% vs. 8%, $p < 0.001$). In conclusion, prevalence and incidence of HCV infection averaged 22.3% and 7.3%, respectively. Our results also suggest that HCV infection is mediated by not only transfusion but also other environmental factors, especially in long-term dialysis patients.

86

Increased Interdialytic Weight Gain is Associated with Better Biochemical Indicies of Nutrition in Chronic Hemodialysis Patient

SN Yun, DC Jin, SJ Ahn, SY Kim, WS Koo, EJ Choi, YS Chang, BK Bang

Department of Internal Medicine, Catholic University Medical College, Seoul, Korea

It had been considered that the interdialytic weight gain in chronic hemodialysis patient was due to water intake. The study was undertaken to determine the effect of interdialytic weight gain on the biochemical indicies of nutrition in the assumption that increased weight gain might be associated with increased food intake as well as increased water ingestion. The 47 patients with maintenance hemodialysis (3 times/week) were classified into two groups according to the percent increase of interdialytic weight gain to dry weight: group 1 ($\geq$5%, n = 20) and group 2 (< 5%, n = 27). The sex, dialysis duration and causes of chronic renal failure were not significantly different between groups but the age (42$\pm$15 in group 1 vs 53$\pm$15 in group 2, p = 0.017) and the dry weight (47.0$\pm$9.4 kg in group 1 vs 57.0$\pm$7.3 kg in group 2, p = 0.0004) were significantly different between groups. The value of predialysis BUN (89.80$\pm$14.99 vs 75.84$\pm$19.93 (mg/dl), p = 0.0118), albumin (4.44$\pm$0.34 vs 4.19$\pm$0.39 (g/dl), p = 0.0307) and Kt/V (1.51$\pm$0.17 vs 1.36$\pm$0.25, p = 0.0297) in group 1 were higher than those in group 2. The value of total protein, cholesterol, triglyceride and NPCR were not significantly different between groups. In conclusion, increased weight gain was associated with better biochemical indicies of nutrition in young patient with adequate dialysis.

87

Body Composition Assessment with Bioelectric Impedance Analysis in Hemodialysis Patients

DC Jin, SY Kim, WS Koo, EJ Choi, YS Chang, BK Bang

Department of Internal Medicine, Catholic University Medical College, Seoul, Korea

The body water gain assessment is one of the most important factor in hemodialysis patient care for prevention of complication, i.e. congestive heart failure. The total body water before and after dialysis and fat composition of maintenance hemodialysis patients were assessed with bioelectric impedance analysis. Total 135 end stage renal disease patients (59 male, 76 female) were enrolled the study (mean hemodialysis duration: 44.0 months, mean dialysis times per week: 2.27). Each of two electrodes were attached on the wrist and ankle for bioelectric impedance measurement with 800μA, 50Hz alternative current and total body water, % fat, fat free weight were calculated. Before the hemodialysis, mean body weight was 61.0$\pm$7.2kg, mean % fat was 13.9$\pm$7.0%, total body water/body weight ratio was 0.646$\pm$0.06 in male patients and 51.7$\pm$8.6kg, 22.0$\pm$7.1%, 0.588$\pm$0.06 in female patients, respectively. After the hemodialysis, mean body weight was 58.5$\pm$7.0kg, mean % of fat was 18.3$\pm$7.8%, total body water/body weight ratio was 0.606$\pm$0.06 in male patients and 49.2$\pm$8.4kg. 27.3$\pm$7.7%, 0.053$\pm$0.06 in female patients, respectively. The reduction of total body water was assessed greater than body water reduction. The bioelectric impedance analysis may be very helpful for assessment of dry weight, weight reduction by ultrafiltration, nutritional status of each hemodialysis patients.

88

Clinical Observation of Liver Disease in Hemodialysis, CAPD and Kidney Transplant Patients

Jee Yoon Kim, Joong Kyoung Kim, Myeong Sun Yoon, Si Rhae Lee

Department of Internal Medicine, Bong Seang Hospital, Pusan, Korea

Hemodialysis (HD), CAPD, and kidney transplant (KTP) patients are at risk of liver disease because of frequent venipuncture, blood transfusion and immunosuppressants. A survey of prevalence and clinical outcome for liver disease was carried out on 88 HD, 230 CAPD, and 222 KTP patients at our hospital using Abbot HBV, anti-HCV EIA.

The mean age (yrs) was 44.7$\pm$1.4 (Mean$\pm$SEM) in HD, 45.1$\pm$0.8 in CAPD and 40.9$\pm$0.7 in KTP. The mean treatment duration (mo) was 32.4$\pm$2.6, 30.4$\pm$1.7 and 55.1$\pm$1.7 in HD, CAPD and KTP respectively. A mean dose of prior blood transfusion was 15.7

(0 ~ 71) units in HD, 4.2 (0 ~ 89) units in CAPD. The HBV positivity was 11.4% (10/88) in HD, 14.4% (33/230) in CAPD and 7.6% (17/222) in KTP. The anti-HCV positivity was 13.6% (12/88) in HD, 7.9% (18/230) in CAPD and 12.2% (27/222) in KTP.

Of 88 HD patients, 21 (23.8%) had liver dysfunction, broken down as follows: 3 out of 10 HBV positive patients (30%), 8 out of 12 anti-HCV positive patients (66.6%) and 10 out of 66 patients without HBV or anti-HCV antibody (15.1%). Of 230 CAPD patients, 31 (13.5%) had liver dysfunction, broken down as follows: 18 out of 33 HBV positive patients (54.5%), 7 out of 18 anti-HCV positive patients (38.9%) and 6 out of 179 patients without HBV or anti-HCV antibody (3.4%). Of 222 KTP patients, 36 (16.2%) had liver dysfunction, broken down as follows : 7 out of 17 HBV positive (41%), 10 out of 17 HBV positive (41%) 10 out of 27 anti-HCV positive patients (37%) and 19 out of 178 patients without HBV or anti-HCV antibody (10.7%).

Of 27 succumbed patients, 10 (11.3%) were noted among 88 HD, 14 (6.1%) among 230 CAPD and 3 (1.3%) among 222 KTP. The causes of death were: cardiovascular in 25.9%, infection 22.2%, hepatic failure 11.1% (3 patients), treatment withdrawal 14.8% and unknown 25.9%. Among the 3 patients who expired due to hepatic failure, 2 were in CAPD, 1 in KTP and none in HD.

In conclusion, the incidence of hepatic dysfunction among the HBV positive patients was significantly higher in CAPD than HD and KTP group. The incidence of hepatic dysfunction among the anti-HCV positive patients was significantly higher in HD than CAPD and KTP groups. We could not find any significant correlation with hepatic death in HD, CAPD or KTP. But further study is needed to figure out possible influence of HBV or HCV infection on the mortality rate with the treatment modalities.

89

Outcome on CAPD after Renal Transplant Failure

T.H. Kwon, Y.L. Kim[a], D.K. Cho[a], Y.W. Kim[b]

[a]Department of Internal Medicine,
[b]Department of Surgery, Kyungpook University Hospital, Taegu, Korea

To assess whether patients failing renal transplant and commencing continuous ambulatory peritoneal dialysis (CAPD) for the treatment of end stage renal disease (ESRD) have high risk of infective and catheter-related complications, we retrospectively reviewed the clinical outcome of 8 patients failing renal transplant and commencing CAPD (Group A). Then, for each of these patients, 16 comparison subjects were chosen from CAPD patients of our hospital; matching variables were age, sex, CAPD duration and underlying disease of ESRD (Group B). In Group A, 8 patients (4 male/4 female) with a mean age of 35 ± 8.9 years had graft survival of 26.5 ± 16.4 months and were treated with CAPD for 31 ± 23.9 months post-transplant. Immunosuppressive agents were not administered after commencement of CAPD. After renal transplant failure, 3 patients developed pancytopenia, 2 had hepatitis B-related chronic liver disease, 1 of whom had gastric ulcer. In Group B, 16 patients (8 male/8 female) with a mean age of 36 ± 10.6 years and were treated CAPD for 31.8 ± 22.9 months. Among them, 3 patients developed hepatitis B-related chronic liver disease. The peritonitis and exit-site infection rates were similar in Group A (1 per 14.7 patient-months/1 per 13.2 patient-months). and Group B (1 per 13.2 patient-months 1 per 36.3 patient-months). The leakage rates were similar. 3/10 catheters developed pericatheter leaks for a percentage rate of 30% in Group A and 3/17 catheters developed pericatheter leaks for a percentage rate of 17.6%. The catheter removal rates were similar in Group A (0.19/patient-year) and Group B (0.09/patient-year). One death was as a result of sepsis 5 months post-CAPD in Group A. Although the small sample size in this study limited definite conclusion, patients commencing CAPD after renal transplant failure had similar infective and catheter-related complications and did not have a particularly poor outcome.

90

CAPD in End-Stage Renal Disease Patients with Preexisting Liver Cirrhosis

Y.L. Kim, T.H. Kwon, D.K. Cho

Department of Internal Medicine, Kyungpook University Hospital, Taegu, Korea

Purpose. The spontaneous tendency to arterial hypotension in cirrhotic patients makes adequate hemodialysis therapy extremely difficult. Hemodialysis in these patients may produce intradialytic hypotension, limiting the amount of ultrafiltration. These patients are also at high risk for gastrointestinal bleeding, which can be exacerbated by anticoagulation. Recently peritoneal dialysis has been suggested for the management of this population.

Patients. Seven patients with chronic renal failure and liver cirrhosis treated by CAPD are described. Six of the seven patients were complicated by ascites on starting CAPD. Hepatocellular carcinoma was identified in one patient. Three had been transferred from hemodialysis for hemodynamic intolerance, one for vascular access problem. All PD catheters were surgically placed.

Results. The hemodynamic tolerance was excellent in all patients. Four patients developed bleeding immediately after catheter insertion. Two patients developed early leaks and one patient late leak. Four patients had a decline in serum albumin level of 0.5 gm/dl or more during the course of chronic PD. Peritonitis occurred on average at 8.6 month interval. Three episodes of catheter removal occurred in 147 patient-months of PD (0.24 per patient-year). Four patients died while maintained on PD; three deaths were due to hepatic encephalopathy on PD for duration of 4 to 60 months and the fourth was due to peritonitis after 24 months of PD. One patient died due to malnutrition after 2 months on switching to hemodialysis because of peritonitis after 32 months of PD.

Conclusion. Early mechanical complications after catheter insertion (bleeding, leak) were more common than usual. But CAPD was better tolerable than hemodialysis and may be a reasonable chronic with an acceptable survival rate in end-stage renal disease patients with preexisting liver cirrhosis.

91

The Risk Factors Associated with Early Death in Patients with Catheter Removal due to Peritonitis

S. Cho, S.J. Kim, M.Y. Paik, J.H. Kim, J.H. Bang, T.H. Kwon, Y.L. Kim, D.K. Cho

Department of Internal Medicine, Kyungpook University Hospital, Taegu, Korea

To evaluate risk factors associated with early death (within 3 months) after catheter removal due to peritonitis, we reviewed 28 patients among 219 CAPD patients between January 1988 and March 1995 in Kyungpook University Hospital. Eight patients died within 3 months after chronic catheter removal (G-1). Fourteen patients had been alive beyond 12 months after catheter removal (G-2). Using Chi-Square analysis, age, sex, CAPD duration, diabetes mellitus, liver cirrhosis, cardiac disease, frequency of peritonitis, etiologic organisms, exit site infection, tunnel infection, abdominal abscess, serum albumin level, serum cholesterol level, duration from final peritonitis to catheter removal were compared. There was increased frequency of liver cirrhosis, cardiac disease, and exit site infection at the time of catheter removal in G-1 compared to G-2 ($p < 0.05$). G-1 tended to have old age, hypoalbuminemia, and hypercholesterolemia compared to G-2 (x^2_{M-H} test for linear association; p = 0.1480/0.0540/0.0965) ; while sex, CAPD duration, diabetes mellitus, frequency of peritonitis, etiologic organisms, tunnel infection, abdominal abscess, or duration from final peritonitis to catheter removal had no significant adverse effects on early death. In summary, the risk factors associated with early death after catheter removal due to peritonitis were liver cirrhosis, cardiac disease, and exit site infection at the time of catheter removal.

92

The Effect of Dialysis Dose on Preservation of Lean Body Mass (LBM) in Continuous Ambulatory Peritoneal Dialysis (CAPD) Patients

S.W. Lee, S.W. Kang, K.H. Choi, H.Y. Lee, D.S. Han

Department of Internal Medicine, Yonsei University College of Medicine, Seoul, Korea

Purpose. Malnutrition has been reported to be as high as 40% in CAPD patients and changes in LBM have been purported to reflect long term nutritional status. To examine the effect of dialysis dose on the preservation of LBM over time in CAPD patients, this study was undertaken.

Methods. We retrospectively analyzed urea kinetic and creatinine excretion data from 31 stable CAPD patients whose first kinetic study was done within 6 months after initiation of CAPD and was followed up every 6 months for more than 1 year. LBM was calculated according to the formula of Keshaviah (JASN, Jan, 1994).

Results. The patients were divided into two groups, group I in whom LBM at 12 month declined more than 5% of 0 month value (n = 14) and group II whose LBM remained unchanged or increased (n = 17). In group I, weekly Kt/V urea at 6 month (2.00 ± 0.41) was similar to 0 month (2.18 ± 0.16) but it decreased significantly at 12 month (1.89 ± 0.38, $p < 0.05$ compared to 0 month). There were no significant changes in weekly Kt/V in group II during the follow-up period (2.23 ± 0.57, 2.17 ± 0.71, 2.07 ± 0.63 at 0, 6, 12 month, respectively). BUN, NPCR, residual renal function, urinary creatinine excretion and weekly Ccr decreased significantly ($p < 0.05$) at 12 month in group I, but not in group II. Serum creatinine and dialysate creatinine excretion increased significantly ($p < 0.05$) at 12 month in group II, but not in group I. BWt, BMI and serum albumin were unchanged in both groups during the follow-up period. When the patients were divided into two groups according to the mean weekly Kt/V over 12 months, the LBM at 12 month as percentage of 0 month decreased significantly (95.0 ± 10.3%, $p < 0.05$) in the patients with low mean weekly Kt/V (n = 16, 1.76 ± 0.23), but in patients with high mean weekly Kt/V (n = 15, 2.45 ± 0.43) the LBM remained unchanged (98.5 ± 12.3%, $p > 0.05$). The mean LBM did not correlated with mean serum albumin, NPCR, residual renal function, weekly Ccr and weekly Kt/V. Mean residual renal function correlated positively with mean weekly Kt/V (r = 0.76) and weekly Ccr (r = 0.88).

Conclusion. The preservation of LBM may be affected by the dialysis dose and it is important to monitor the dialysis dose and LBM in CAPD patients regularly because modification of dialysis dose may prevent this loss of LBM.

93

The Evolution of Hepatitis C Virus (HCV) Infection According to The Mode of Dialysis in Patients with End Stage Renal Disease (ESRD)

S.W. Lee, S.W. Kang, K.H. Choi, H.Y. Lee, D.S. Han

Department of Internal Medicine, Yonsei University College of Medicine, Seoul, Korea

Purpose. HCV infection is highly prevalent in patients with ESRD treated in dialysis units, but there have been few reports about the transition of viremia and incidence of chronic hepatitis according to the mode of dialysis in Korea. To investigate the effect of mode of dialysis (HD and CAPD) on viremia and liver function in dialysis patients, this study was undertaken.

Methods. We examined prospectively HCV-RNA and liver function in anti-HCV positive ESRD patients every three months for one year. Anti-HCV was tested by second-generation anti-HCV enzyme immunoassay and HCV-RNA was detected by polymerase chain reaction.

Results. The HD and CAPD patients were 53 and 364, respectively. Anti-HCV positive patients were 23 (12 in HD, 11 in CAPD), whose mean ages were 53.4 ± 14.0 years, 56.5% were male, and median duration of dialysis was 74.9 (27.3-137.3) months. One patient on HD and two patients on CAPD expired due to sepsis. Seroconversion to anti-HCV positive was noted in two cases (2/41, 4.9%) of HD but none in CAPD among the anti-HCV negative ESRD patients. Two CAPD patients were switched to HD due to fungal peritonitis. The incidence of anti-HCV positive patients was significantly higher in HD with 22.6% (12/53) compared to 3.0% (11/364) in CAPD ($p < 0.05$). Between HD and CAPD, no significant differences were noted in the incidence and number of transfusion, serum ALT, ferritin, γGTP, the positivity of anti-HCV, the incidence of chronic hepatitis (16.7 vs 18.2%) and the positivity of HCV-RNA (88.3 vs 90.0%) except the duration of dialysis (109.8 vs 58.2 months, $p < 0.05$). Of these 23, HCV-RNA positive (n = 20) and negative (n = 3) group showed no significant difference in the incidence and number of transfusion, mode of dialysis, and the incidence of chronic hepatitis, serum ferritin, γGTP, and the positivity of anti-HBc, except in serum AST (27.2 ± 22.3 vs 7.0 ± 3.0 IU/L, $p < 0.05$) and ALT (35.0 ± 27.6 vs 7.0 ± 3.0 IU/L, $p < 0.05$).

Conclusions. The incidence of anti-HCV positive patients was significantly higher in HD and abnormal liver function was frequently observed in HCV-RNA positive patients. But the positivity of HCV-RNA and the incidence of chronic hepatitis were not significantly different according to the mode of dialysis. A long term study may by needed to find a more beneficial mode of dialysis to maintain normal liver function in HCV-RNA positive patients.

94

Correlation between Nutritional Status and Urea Kinetic Modeling in Hemodialysis Patients

M.K. Song[a], S.W. Lee, S.W. Kang[a], K.H. Choi[a], H.Y. Lee[a], D.S. Han[a], J.H. Lee[b], M.K. Cho[b]

[a]Department of Internal Medicine, Yonsei University College of Medicine,
[b]Department of Food Nutrition, Yonsei University College of Human Ecology, Seoul, Korea

Purpose. Protein-calorie malnutrition is a common problem in patients undergoing maintenance hemodialysis due to multiple factors. It is well known that optimal nutritional support and adequacy of hemodialysis are the most important factors to determine the morbidity and mortality of these patients. To investigate the relationship between nutritional status and dialysis adequacy in hemodialysis patients, this study was undertaken.

Methods. Nutritional status was assessed by subjective global assessment (SGA) and dietary food intake by 24 hour recall method as well as by anthropometric measurement in 82 stable hemodialysis patients. Individual nutritional status was compared with various biochemical and urea kinetic variables such as normalized protein catabolic rate (NPCR), Kt/V and standardized creatinine clearnace (SCCr).

Results. There were 57 men and 25 women with mean hemodialysis duration of 30.5 months and the most common causative disease was chronic glomerulonephritis (57.2%). The mean concentration of albumin was 4.3±0.4 g/dl, NPCR 1.04±0.24 g/kg/day, delivered Kt/V_{urea} 1.30±0.31 and SCCr 66.56±10.69 $l/wk/1.73m^2$. Thirteen patients (15.9%) were classified as malnourished by SGA. Malnourished patients had significantly longer hemodialysis duration (27.0 vs 48.9 months) and lower values in blood urea nitrogen concentration (80.4±18.0 vs 59.5±19.1mg/dl), RRF (residual renal function) (1.21 vs 0.31 ml/min), NPCR (1.09±0.22 vs 0.77±0.14 g/kg/day) and Kt/V_{urea} (1.33 ±0.31 vs 1.15±0.28) compared to the well-nourished patients. NPCR showed no correlation with serum albumin value, total body muscle, lean body mass and Kt/V_{urea}. But it revealed a weak positive correlation with RRF, TW-Kt/V (total weekly Kt/V_{urea}) and TWR-Kt/V (total weekly Kt/V_{urea} including RRF).

Conclusion. In conclusion, nutritional support and adequate dialysis should be emphasized in patients with longer hemodialysis duration and lower blood urea nitrogen. NPCR and Kt/V_{urea} appear to be a more sensitive measure of nutritional status assessed by SGA in hemodialysis patients than anthropometry and other biochemical parameters such as serum albumin. Therefore regular follow-up of NPCR and Kt/V_{urea} with an adequate adjustment of dialysis prescription may contribute to improve the nutritional status of patients. Further prospective study is needed to evaluate the exact relationship between dialysis dose and nutritional status of hemodialysis patients.

95

Effect of Hemoperfusion on Treatment for Paraquat Intoxication

K.Y. Lee, T.H. Lee

Nephrology Division, Department of Internal Medicine, Presbyterian Medical Center, Chonju, Korea

Paraquat is a very potent herbicide which causes fatal toxicity when ingested, and there is no specific antidote against it. So it is known that most of the patients who ingested it die of pulmonary fibrosis. We used hemoperfusion (HP) for the treatment against paraquat poisoning from July 1993 till March 1994 and analyzed the data using SPSS/PC ver. 4.0 for chi-square and t-test for mean±SD. The results were as follows; (1) A total of 36 paraquat poisoning patients (22 males and 14 females, mean age 48.8 years) visited our hospital, and 18 patients out of 36 received hemoperfusion (total 90 cycles) ; there was statistically significant difference in ages (41.4±15.6 year vs. 56.2±15.0 year, $p < 0.05$), but there was no significant difference in the amount of paraquat ingested (59.9±72.7ml vs. 78.6±83.6ml, NS), gastric lavages (13/18 vs. 16/18, NS), and use of Fuller's earth (8/18 vs. 4/18, NS) between the patients who received HP and those who did not receive HP. (2) All the patients who did not receive HP died, but 9 patients out of 18 who received HP survived ($p < 0.005$). There was no significant difference in ages (46.8±9.8 year vs. 36.0±18.8 year, NS), amount of paraquat ingested (87.5±94.2ml vs. 34.8±36.4ml, NS), gastric lavages (7/9 vs. 6/9, NS), use of Fuller's earth (5/9 vs. 3/9, NS) and interval from the ingestion of paraquat to HP (52.4±49.9 hr vs. 38.3±39.7 hr, NS) between patients who died and those who survived, but Scr levels on arrival in expired patients were higher than those in surviving patients (5.0±3.5mg/dl vs. 1.4±

0.6mg/dl, $p < 0.05$). Therefore, this suggests that HP is very effective in the treatment of paraquat poisoning, and HP is the most important factor in the prognosis of the patients.

96

Clinical Study of Continuous Ambulatory Peritoneal Dialysis in Children

Won-Kyu Choi, Min-Joong Kwon, Pyung-Kil Kim

Department of Pediatrics, Yonsei University College of Medicine, Seoul, Korea

CAPD has established itself as an alternative therapeutic modality to hemodialysis in the treatment of patients with end-stage renal disease. Especially in children, many of the advantages originally reported with the use of CAPD have been reported with large population studies. This includes easy of training and management, no requirement of repetitive venipuncture, less restriction of diet, stable salt and water balance easy of blood pressure control. Clinical studies carried out on the 29 cases of CAPD who had been treated from November 1985 to February 1995. The following results were obtained: Nineteen cases were males and ten cases were females, with male to female ratio of 1.9:1. The mean age of the patients was 12.9 ± 3.1 years old. The original renal diseases of ESRD were proven in 22 cases. The common renal disesaes were reflux nephropathy and chronic glomerulonephritis each in 4 cases. Other diseases were focal segmental glomerulosclerosis in 3 cases, Henoch-Schönlein purpura nephritis in 2 cases, hemolytic uremic syndrome in 2 cases, and Alport syndrome, Ig A nephropathy and lupus nephritis were followed. The mean duration of CAPD was 16.1 ± 19.9 months. Peritonitis was most common complication whose incidence was one episode/patient/7.6 months. Other complications were exit site infection in 3 cases, obstruction in 3 cases, and leakage of dialysate in 3 cases, peritoneal adhesion, malposition and scrotal swelling were followed. The most common etiologic organisms of peritonitis was staphyococcus coagulase negative in 8 cases and staphylococcus aureus was followed. Others were pseudomonas, Enterococcus species and E. coli. As increasing renal transplantation, CAPD in children has been more important as renal replacement therapy. Although the pathophysiologic studies of patient on CAPD has been performed, more additive researches must be followed.

97

Penetration of Exotoxin-A Related Cytokine-Inducing Substances through Dialyzer Membranes

Steffen Krautzig, Gerhard Lonnemann, Karl M, Koch

Department of Nephrology, Medizinische Hochschule Hannover, Germany

Gram negative microorganisms such as Pseudomonas species are routinely found in dialysate. These bacteria release cytokine-inducing substances including lipopolysaccharides (LPS), peptidoglycans and exotoxins. In contrast to the LAL assay which is specific for LPS, human mononuclear cells (PBMC) produce cytokines such as interleukin-1 (IL-1) in response to all pyrogens including exotoxins. Recent in vitro and in vivo data clearly show that intact dialyzer membranes are permeable to PBMC-activating bacteria-derived pyrogens. However, the use of the in vitro PBMC incubation as a test system in combination with the LPS specific antibiotic polymyxin B (PmxB) revealed that predominantly non-LPS related pyrogens penetrate dialyzer membranes. We now performed in vitro experiments using a goat antiserum raised against exotoxin A from Pseudomonas aeruginosa in the PBMC culture to further analyze the IL-1-inducing activity penetrating dialyzer membranes. Polyamide membranes ($n = 6$) were challenged with increasing doses of a culture filtrate of P. aeruginosa (PA 103) grown in bicarbonate dialysate. Dilutions of the challenge material (pre filter) as well as the filtrate (post filter) were incubated with human donor PBMC in the presence and absence of PmxB, and a combination of PmxB with the exotoxin A antiserum (anti exo A). IL-1β was measured by radioimmunoassay in PBMC lysates after 18 hours of incubation. The results (mean $\pm$ SEM) show that the IL-1β -inducing activity of the pre filter samples (23 ± 2 ng/ml) was reduced by PmxB to 18 ± 2 ng/ml ($p < 0.05$) and by PmxB+anti exo A to 11 ± 1.5 ng/ml ($p < 0.01$). The IL-1-inducing activity in the post filter samples (7.5 ± 1 ng/ml) was not reduced by PmxB (7.6 ± 0.8 ng/ml) but reduced by PmxB+anti exo A to 2.5 ± 0.5 ng/ml ($p < 0.01$). We conclude that exotoxin A and/or fragments thereof participate in the pyrogenic activity penetrating dialyzer membranes.

98

Simple Models for Fluid Transport during Peritoneal Dialysis

Jacek Waniewski, Olof Heimbürger, Andrzej Werynski, Bengt Lindholm

Karolinska Institute, Stockholm, Sweden, and Institute of Biocybernetics and Biomedical Engineering, Warsaw, Poland

Peritoneal fluid transport can be predicted using different simplified formulas. To evaluate three such models, fluid transport was studied in 38 single six hour dwell studies using standard glucose 1.36%, 2.27% and 3.86% dialysis fluids in 33 patients on continuous ambulatory peritoneal dialysis (CAPD). Dialysate volume and the peritoneal reabsorption rate were measured using radioiodinated serum albumin (RISA) as a marker. The dialysate volume over dwell time curves were examined using three mathematical models of fluid transport for solutions with a crystalloid osmotic agent: Model P based on phenomenologically derived exponential function of time (Pyle, 1981)

$Qv\ (t) = A_p exp\ (-kpt)\ -bp$

Model OS based on linear relationship between the rate of net volume change, Qv, to the difference of osmolality in dialyate and blood, $\triangle$OS,

$Qv = a_{os} \triangle OS - b_{OS}$

and Model G based on linear relationship between Qv and the difference of glucose concentration in dialysate and blood, $\triangle$CG,

$Qv = a_G \triangle C_G - b_G$

All three models provided a good description of the measured dialysate volume over time curves, however the descriptions with Models OS and G for glucose 3.86% fluid were slightly but significantly less precise. The coefficients of Model OS were stable in time, but the coefficients of Models G and P depended in general on the time period used for their estimation, especially for glucose 3.86% dialysis fluid. The evaluation of a separate series of eight dwell studies with solutions containing amino acids 2.70% (instead of glucose) as osmotic agent, using Models OS and P, showed that the transport coefficients were stable in time and both models provided equally percise description. These results suggested that all three models can be used but models P and OS can be preferred for practical applications such as predictions of fluid transport with alternative cristalloid osmotic agents. Furthermore, we found that the peritoneal barrier for fluid transport may change transiently during exchanges with the standard glucose-based dialysis fluid, whereas such changes were not observed with the amino acid-based fluid. This discrepancy may be due to different composition of the dialysis fluids, including osmotic agent, buffer and pH.

99

Interferon Treatment for Chronic Hemodialysis Patients with Chronic Hepatitis C

Fumiaki Marumo

Second Department of Internal Medicine, Faculty of Medicine, Tokyo Medical and Dental University, Bunkyo-ku, Tokyo 113, Japan

High prevalence of hepatitis C virus (HCV) infection has been reported in chronic hemodialysis (HD) patients. Although the occurrence of hepatocellular carcinoma (HCC) has been well known as a clinical outcome of chronic HCV infection, the incidence of HCC has not been investigated in HD patients with HCV infection. Among 2,123 HD patients, 399 patients were positive for serum HCV-antibodies (18.8%), and we experienced 10 patients with HCC during the two years of observation period. HCC was discovered by elevated serum alpha-fetoprotein levels, by autopsy, or by ultrasonography for periodic screening. Although pathological examinations of the liver revealed cirrhosis of chronic active hepatitis in six cases, their liver function tests including serum levels of aminotransferases, albumin, and total bilirubin, and prothrombin time were almost normal. Percentage of prothrombin time in the HD patients with HCC was significantly higher than that of non-HD patients with HCC. These findings indicate the necessity of appropriate treatment for HD patients with HCV infection. Liver biopsy was carried out under peritoneoscopy in chronic HD patients with positive anti-HCV antibodies and increased serum levels of aminotransferases. They were proven to have chronic hepatitis. Then, interferon (IFN) alpha 2b was administered at a dose of 300-600 million units (MU) intramuscularly everyday for 2 wk, and then thrice a week for 22 wk. Blood levels of IFN were measured in the patients and in the controls who received IFN for the treatment of chronic hepatitis C. The Cmax and the AUC in HD patients who received 3 MU of IFN were comparable with those in controls who received 6 MU of IFN. Furthermore, blood half-life of IFN was doubled in HD patients. Although side effects of IFN, including high fever, depression, and consciousness disturbance, were easy to appear in HD patients, careful choice of dose and administration schedule will decrease the incidence of these side effects. Virological prediction of the effectiveness of IFN treatment in HD patients will also be discussed.

improve appetite (erythropoietin) and anabolism (growth hormone and IGF-1). Some preliminary studies suggest that positive nitrogen balance may be obtained with recombinant growth hormone and recombinant IGF-1 in malnourished MD patients. However, larger scale randomized studies need to be performed in order to confirm the efficacy of these treatments in malnourished MD patients.

100

Interventions for Malnutrition in Patients undergoing Maintenance Dialysis

Denis Fouque

Department of Nephrology, Hôpital E. Herriot and University Claude Bernard, Lyon, France

Patients undergoing maintenance dialysis (MD) frequently manifest mild to severe malnutrition, a fact reported to begin before the onset of dialysis. Despite intensive counseling, MD patients often cannot improve their nutritional status.

This condition might be partly explained by psychological as well as metabolic factors. Food intake is often reduced by anorexia. A state of persistant catabolism has been reported in these patients, and may be caused by chronic acidosis, impaired pharmacokinetics and resistance for anabolic factors such as growth hormone, insulin and insulin-like growth factor (IGF) -1. Losses of nutrients including glucose, amino acid and vitarmins occur during the dialysis treatment. Negative nitrogen balance has been reported during the hemodialysis procedure. In certain conditions, reuse of dialyzers are associated with an increase in albumin losses into dialysate and a decrease in serum albumin in MHD patients. Thus, a chronic imbalance between protein synthesis and degradation and, hence, muscle mass, may be present in MD patients.

Intradialytic parenteral nutrition has been used when oral supplements have failed to improve patients nutritional status. Lipids infusion alone or a all-in-one solution containing glucose, lipids and amino acids have been administered to malnourished MHD patients with encouraging result. Enrichment of hemodialysate with glucose or amino acid have been reported to induce a positive balance in the corresponding compound. The use of amino acid infusion in the peritoneal cavity is associated with a more positive nitrogen balance in malnourished CPD patients. Growth factors may

101

The Influence of Repeated Plasma Exchange on Plasme Levels of Inflammatory Cytokines

V. Tesař[a], E. Jelinková[a], Z. Mašek[b], J. Lachmanová[a], I. Rychlik[a], J. Žabka[a], M. Merta[a], A. Stejskalová[c]

[a]lst Department of Medicine, [b]3rd Department of Medicine, [c]Department of Pathology, Charles University, Prague, Czech Republic Supported by grant of MH No. 2228-3

Plasma exchange (PE) may be used as an effective treatment of some patients with active renal vasculitis and/or lupus nephritis. To evaluate the influence of repeated PE (5 sessions) on the activation of some proinflammatory (IL-6, IL-8, IL-1ß) and anti-inflammatory (IL-1ra) cytokines we measured using ELISA concentrations of these cytokines in plasma-filtrates and in the samples of plasma taken before and after each session of PE in a small group of 13 patients (pts) with autoimmune disease with bioptically proven kidney involvement (10 with ANCA-vascultitis with crescentic nephritis, remaining 3 with active lupus nephritis). All these pts were concomitantly treated by combined immunousuppression with corticosteroids and cyclophosphamide.

Plasma IL-1ra (from 909.0 ± 964.02 to 1437.41 ± 1323.11pg/ml, $p < 0.01$) and plasma IL-6 (from 33.72 ± 71.82 to 55.12 ± 99.19pg/ml, $p < 0.05$) increased significantly during sessions of PE, but plasma IL-8 increased only during the first PE session and IL-1ß did not change at all. Levels of IL-6, IL-1ß and IL-1ra were significantly lower in plasmafiltrate than in plasma after PE.

On the basis of plasma levels of IL-1ra in the beginning of the treatment patients could be subdivided into two group: 1) 7pts with low levels of IL-1ra not different from controls (345.3 ± 123.4 pg/ml) -low cytokine group (LC), 2) 6pts with high levels of IL1ra significantly higher than controls (1997.8 ± 1398.6 vs. 316.4 ± 48.3 pg/ml, $p < 0.01$-high cytokine group-HC). HC pts had also in comparison with controls significantly increased plasma levels of IL-6 (100.0 ± 147.3 vs. 2.7 ± 0.85 pg/ml. $p < 0.05$), IL-8 (101.2 ± 29.7 vs. 30.2 ± 4.55 pg/ml, $p < 0.001$) and IL-1ß (3.15 ± 0.35 vs. 2.8 ± 0.08 pg/ml, $p < 0.01$).

Plasma IL-1ra significantly decreased during 5 sessions of PE only in pts with high plasma IL-1ra (from 1977.8 ± 1398.6 to 944.3 ± 520.4 pg/ml, $p < 0.05$), but neither plasma IL-6, IL-8 nor IL-1ß changed significantly.

There was no important difference in plasma creatinine and histological severity between HC and LC pts. In time of diagnosis 4 out of 6 HC pts and 3 out of 7LC patients had to be dialyze. In the HC group 2 pts died and 1 pt with previously preserved renal function had to be regularly dialyzed. In the LC group 1 pt died, but renal function was restored in all three previously dialyzed pts.

In conclusion, pts with active renal vasculitis and lupus nephritis could be subdivided on the basis of the plasma levels of proinflammatory cytokines and IL-1ra into low cytokine and high cytokine group. High or low plasma levels of inflammatory cytokines could not be predicted on the basis of renal biopsy or renal function and their significance for the prognosis of these pts is unclear. Plasma IL-1ra decreased during repeated sessions of PE in high cytokine group despite increase of its plasma levels after each plasma session.

102

Hypolipidemic Effect of Apherent Therapy on Aggregation Ability of Atherogenic Liporoteins

Tarabrin Alexander

Institute of Surgery, Irkutsk, Russia

Hypolipidemic effect of apherent therapy (hemosorption, plasmapheresis) on aggregation ability of atherogenic lipoproteins (LP) was studied.

Time parameters of the rate of heparin-induced aggregation of summary atherogenic LP (LDL, VLDL) and lipid level were determined in blood serum samples obtained from hyperlipidemic patients prior to and following hemosorption (21 pts) and plasmapheresis (15pts). Aggregation rate was determined at register photometer through changes in optical density (OD, 364-365nm) after adding heparin (50mcl, 1000U/ml) to the medium, containing 50 mcl of blood serum in 1ml 25mmol $CaCl_2$. Two time parameters were detected on aggregation curve: T_1-the end of first aggregation phase manifested as OD maximum; T_2-the beginning of the second aggregation phase (large aggregates formation) manifested as OD lowering.

Results. We observed the decrease in total cholesterol by 16% and 23%, in triglycerides by 38% and 21%, in phospholipids by 16% and 15%, in total lipids by 21% and 19% in hemosorption and plasmapheresis group respectively. It was accompanied by increase in both time parameters: T_1 from 3.2 ± 0.27 to 4.6 ± 0.42min, $p < 0.05$ and T_2 from 6.0 ± 0.40 to 8.1 ± 0.69min, $p < 0.05$ in hemosorption group; T_1 from 3.6 ± 0.23 to 4.9 ± 0.62min, $p < 0.05$ and T_2 from 5.7 ± 0.30 to 7.8 ± 1.17min, $p < 0.05$ in plasmapheresis group.

Conclusion. Hypolipidemic effect of apherent therapy is paralleled by the decrease in aggregation ability of atherogenic LP. We consider it to be an additional positive effect of apherent method which provides for the prevention of LP fixation and accumulation in the vessel wall.

103

Clearance of Serum Middle Molecule Peptide as the Index of the Efficacy of Apherent Therapy in Ischemic Patients

I. Rudykh, E. Kuznetsova. V. Leontieva, T. Kurilskaya, A. Runovich

Institue of Surgery, Irkutsk, Russia

The dynamics of middle molecule peptide (MMP) level was studied by HPLC method to assess the effect of apherent therapy in complex treatment of patients with IHD caused by stenotic coronary atherosclerosis.

Blood serum of ischemic patients contained peptide with molecular mass 1000D in the content 7 to 40mcg/ml. The content correlated with the degree of coronary bed affection and clinical severity resulted from previous myocardial infarction and concomitant hypertension. MMP level depended neither on age, nor sex, nor the length of a disease.

Because of drug resistance, 50 pts experienced hemosorption and 40 pts-plasmapheresis. Both procedures influenced the MMP clearance in one way. MMP level decreased by 36.2% following hemosorption, and by 44% following plasmapheresis. The clinical status was improved, as exemplified by reduction in angina events, angina severity, drug taking, also by improving functional indices in exercise testing.

The most marked clinical effect and significant decrease in MMP level was shown in patients of III-IV NYHA class with high initial serum MMP level. Improvement of functional indices was less expressed in moderate coronary failure compared to severe IHD. Accordingly, changes in MMP clearance were less pronounced in the first case. As for the late results serum peptide level was increasing more intensively in patients experienced hemosorption.

Hence, hemosorption and plasmapheresis in complex treatment of patients with severe drug-resistant IHD provides rapid elimination of MMP, thus promoting the improvement in clinical status of patients.

104
Islet Cell Encapsulation

G. Reach

INSERM U341, Diabetes Department, Hôtel-Dieu Hospital, Paris, France

The bioartificial pancreas, in which isolated islets of Langerhans are immunoisolated in an artificial membrane represents a machine which is at the frontier between the worlds of tissue transplantation and artificial organs. Several approaches are possible: Vascular devices, in which blood of the host circulates in contact of a membrane (for instance through a semi-permeable hollow fibre), the islets being placed on its other side in a closed compartment, would be very similar to a hemodialysers, the 'dialysate' compartment containing the islets being closed. Simpler systems, referred to as extravascular systems, including diffusion chambers, microencapsulated islets, or islets placed inside a hollow fibre, may be implanted inside the peritoneal cavity or in the subcutaneous tissue. There is no doubt that some of these systems were able to correct diabetes in animals, although most of the studies were performed in small laboratory animals. The scaling up of these systems remains a major issue, and it is not at all proved that it will not generate new, unexpected problems. For instance, it may be possible that an individual fibre containing islets is able to correct diabetes in a mouse, but that the geometry required to form an implantable 10 meter long fiber would yield a device in which the supply of oxygen and nutrients to all the islets placed in it would be problematic if the system is not richly neovascularized, leading to the concept of bioartificial organoid. On the other hand, it will be necessary to demonstrate the complete safety of the system. Obviously, application to human medicine of these concepts will represent a field for a major bioethical debate.

Author Index

Numbers refer to Abstract No. in the special issue '13th Annual Meeting of the International Society of Blood Purification'